EDiR - The Essential Guide

Judith Babar

Oğuz Dicle

Hildo J. Lamb

Laura Oleaga

Fermín Sáez

EDiR - The Essential Guide

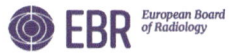

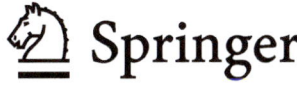

Judith Babar
NHS Foundation Trust
Department of Radiology
Cambridge University Hospitals
Cambridge, United Kingdom

Hildo J. Lamb
Department of Radiology
Leiden University Medical Center
Leiden, The Netherlands

Fermín Sáez
Department of Pediatric Radiology
Hospital Universitario Cruces
UPV-EHU
Barakaldo, Spain

Oğuz Dicle
School of Medicine
Department of Radiology
Dokuz Eylül University
Balçova, Turkey

Laura Oleaga
Radiology
Hospital Clinic of Barcelona
Barcelona, Spain

ISBN 978-3-030-20068-8   ISBN 978-3-030-20066-4   (eBook)
https://doi.org/10.1007/978-3-030-20066-4

This Springer imprint is published by the registered company Springer Nature Switzerland AG
The registered company address is: Gewerbestrasse 11, 6330 Cham, Switzerland

Foreword

I am very pleased to present the EDiR book.

The European Diploma in Radiology (EDiR) was created to provide the radiologists with a certification of excellence, guaranteeing that the holder has a level of knowledge and competence in line with the ESR European Training Curriculum for Radiology. EDiR provides an added value to your CV.

Naturally, we would like all our EDiR candidates to pass the exam. Therefore, we have designed this concise handbook to provide guidance when preparing for the EBR European Diploma in Radiology.

The book contains practical tips, cases, multiple-choice questions and links to EDiR prep sessions. In addition, we have included an overview of safety procedures, as the exam contains safety questions regarding radiation, contrast use, ultrasound, CT, MRI and interventional procedures. There is also a chapter on the principles underlying imaging techniques and processing to prepare you for questions on X-ray, ultrasound, CT, MRI and PET. Last but not the least, there is a chapter on management, as your knowledge in this area will also be tested during the examination.

As a modern society, the ESR would like to provide an increasing amount of online content for our members. We want to ensure that knowledge is available to everyone and everywhere in the world and to guarantee the best possible standards for our specialty, harmonising the level of radiology training within Europe and beyond.

I hope you will find the content of this book a valuable resource and that you will soon be a proud holder of the European Diploma in Radiology!

Finally, I would like to thank Prof. Laura Oleaga and her team of authors for their time, effort and valuable contributions to this book.

Bernd Hamm
Chairman of the ESR Board of Directors (March 2018–March 2019)
Berlin, Germany

Preface

This book was designed by the members of the European Board of Radiology (EBR), the organisation that awards the European Diploma in Radiology (EDiR). It is meant to serve as a precise, effective guide for candidates preparing for the EDiR examination.

EDiR is an international certification method jointly established by the European Society of Radiology and the European Union of Medical Specialists (UEMS, Union Européenne Des Médicins Spécialistes) that opens up a range of opportunities for radiologists developing their professional career. EDiR holders obtain a certificate of excellence and a guarantee that their knowledge and competence is in harmony with the European Training Curriculum (ETC).

The book content has been selected and supervised by the members of several EDiR committees involved in its creation. It includes 13 categories evaluated in the European radiology examination:
1. Abdominal radiology
2. Breast radiology
3. Cardiac radiology
4. Chest radiology
5. Genitourinary radiology
6. Head and neck radiology
7. Interventional and vascular radiology
8. Musculoskeletal radiology
9. Neuroradiology
10. Paediatric radiology
11. Contrast media and radiopharmaceuticals
12. Imaging physics
13. Safety and management

Each chapter is structured in three sections, similar to those in the European examination: first, a section with multiple-choice questions; second, a section with short cases; and third, a section with cases requiring clinical reasoning.

The book also provides chapterwise links to online educational content selected from the ESR Education on Demand platform, as well as relevant references related to each category.

We hope that this book, resulting from the efforts of the members of the EDiR committees and the EBR staff, will contribute to facilitate teaching in radiology and will be a useful training tool for EDiR candidates.

EDiR Book (How to Use It)

How to Use This Book?

Please note that the answers to the questions, the differential diagnosis and the final diagnosis for the cases are provided at the end of each chapter. The book includes links to access additional EDiR preparatory material, as online educational content selected from the ESR Education on Demand Platform as well as relevant literature for each of the categories. References and links appear at the end of each chapter.

As to the references for each of the subspecialties, the first three are on anatomy and congenital lesions, and the following five are on disease.

Judith Babar
Cambridge, UK

Oğuz Dicle
Balçova, Turkey

Hildo J. Lamb
Leiden, The Netherlands

Laura Oleaga
Barcelona, Spain

Fermín Sáez
Barakaldo, Spain

Acknowledgements

We would like to thank all the contributing EDiR committee members for their dedication and work during the long and complex process of writing this book. Their expertise in each of the areas covered was essential, and because of them, the knowledge imparted will cross barriers and benefit future radiologists during their training period. We would also like to extend our thanks particularly to our two coordinators, Prof. Jean-François Chateil and Prof. Mustafa Secil, for their commitment to education and their desire to provide top-quality material through attentive overseeing open to any eventuality. In this line, we cannot miss the opportunity to thank Prof. Carmel J. Caruana for writing the chapters on safety and the technical aspects of radiology, a highly complex task.

We wish to make special mention of our EBR Shareholders' Board for their vote of confidence right from the beginning. Without them, it would have been impossible to launch this important project.

In addition, we would like to express our sincere gratitude to Stefanie Bolldorf and Isabella Weidinger of the ESR office and, most especially, to the chair of the e-Learning Subcommittee, Dr. Sue Barter, for their unerring support at all times. Thanks to them and to the contributors to the ESR Education on Demand Platform, we are able to provide the EDiR Community with access to this valuable material.

We cannot end this section of special mentions without thanking the Springer publishing house for having accepted the challenge of publishing such an innovative book in this area, as well as Ms. Antonella Cerri for guiding us through the production process.

Finally, we would like to dedicate this book to the entire EDiR Community, as they were the inspiration for this project from the planning stage and throughout its development.

Last but not least, we would like to express our gratitude to the following experts that have supported us with their valuable suggestions throughout the preparation of the final content of this guide to the EDiR examination:

- Miraude Adriaensen
- Raffaella Basilico
- Minerva Becker
- Monika Bekiesinska-Figatowska
- Michele Bertolotto
- Carmel J. Caruana
- Filipe Caseiro-Alves

- Eva Castañer
- Jean-François Chateil
- Marcin Czarniecki
- Mukaddes Gümüştekin
- Sven Haller
- Fleur Kilburn-Toppin
- Karl-Friedrich Kreitner
- Winnifred van Lankeren
- Ioana G. Lupescu
- Michael Maher
- Carmen Martínez
- Bogdan Olteanu
- Chantal van Ongeval
- Frank A. Pameijer
- Anagha P. Parkar
- Roar Pedersen
- Jean-Baptiste Pialat
- Maria Raissaki
- Philip Robinson
- Mustafa Secil
- Raman Uberoi
- Meike W. Vernooij
- Stefan Wirth
- Giulia Zamboni

Contents

Abdominal Radiology

Electronic supplementary material The online version of this chapter (https://doi.org/10.1007/978-3-030-20066-4_1) contains supplementary material, which is available to authorized users.

1

Multiple Response Questions (MRQs)

? **MRQ 1**

Regarding liver segment anatomy:

The boundary between segments 6 and 7 is built by which anatomic structures?

(Multiple answers might be correct.)

1. Right portal vein
2. Middle hepatic vein
3. Right hepatic vein
4. Gallbladder fossa
5. Left hepatic vein

? **MRQ 2**

A 32-year-old male with dysphagia:

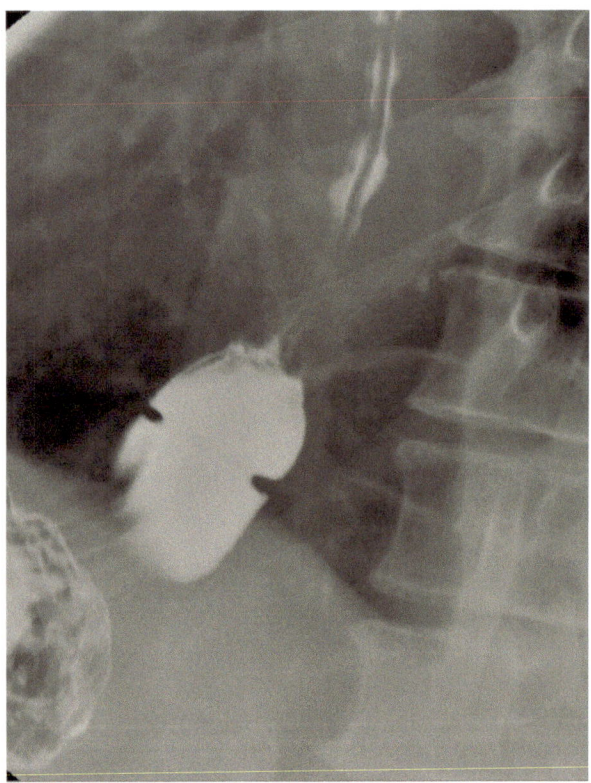

What is the most likely diagnosis?

(Only one option is correct.)

1. Lye stricture
2. Schatzki ring
3. Reflux oesophagitis
4. Squamous cell cancer
5. Normal finding

MRQ 3
Regarding tumour response criteria in oncologic imaging according to RECIST how are liver metastases measured?
(Only one option is correct.)
1. Bi-dimensional measurement of two target lesions
2. The sum of the longest diameters of two target lesions
3. The sum of the longest diameters of five target lesions
4. The longest diameter of the largest lesion
5. The shortest diameter of the largest lesion

MRQ 4
A 66-year-old male presented with recurrent jaundice after cholecystectomy:

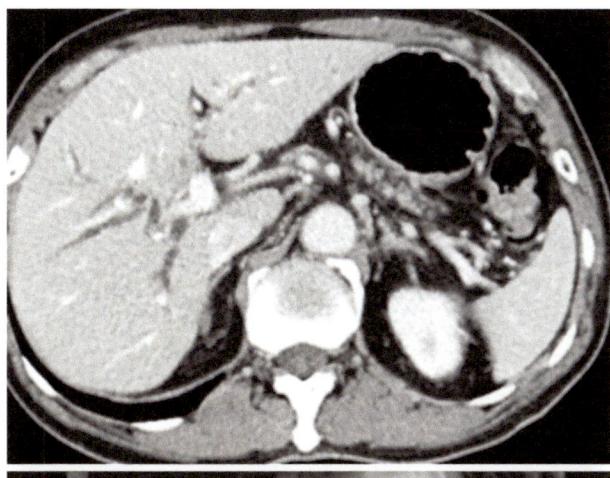

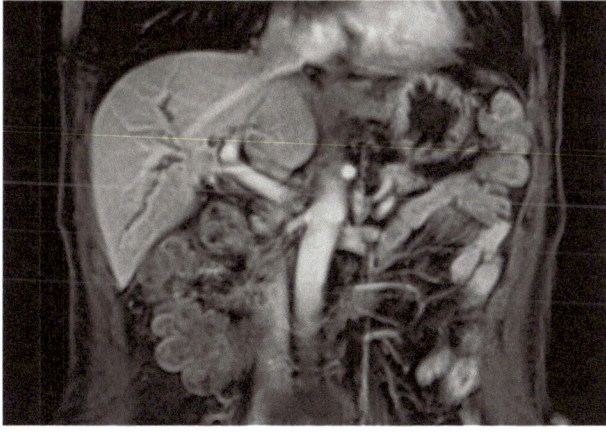

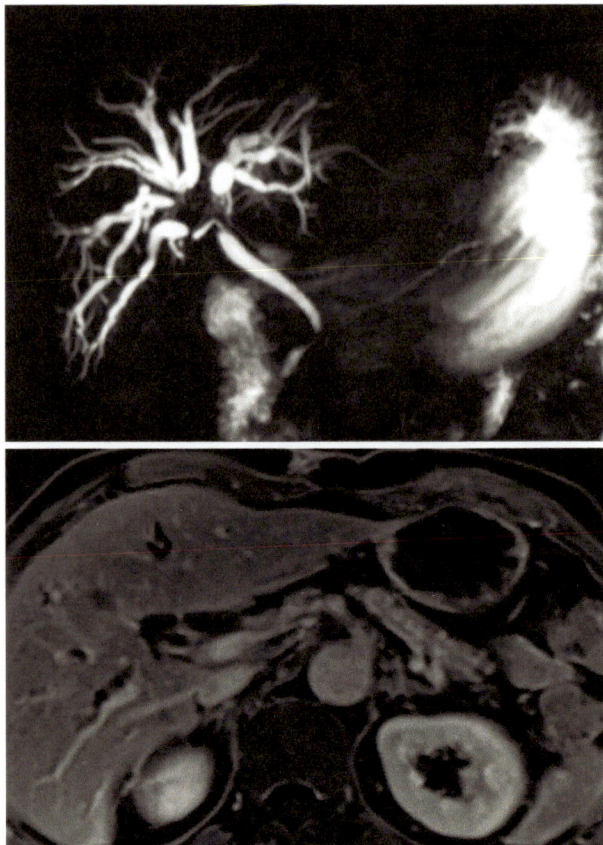

What is the most likely diagnosis?
(Only one option is correct.)
1. Hilar cancer
2. Primary biliary cirrhosis
3. IgG4-related sclerosing cholangitis
4. Pancreatic cancer
5. Intrahepatic stone disease

❓ MRQ 5
Regarding radiation enteritis, which of the following statements are correct?
(Multiple answers might be correct.)
1. It can affect 5–15% of patients treated with radiotherapy
2. It can affect 80% of patients treated with radiotherapy
3. At Small Bowel Series in acute radiation enteritis, the bowel loops appear spastic with luminal narrowing and oedema of mucosal folds
4. At Small Bowel Series in acute radiation enteritis, the bowel loops appear dilated with luminal narrowing and disappearance of mucosal folds
5. Acute radiation enteritis does not show any finding in Small Bowel Series

❓ MRQ 6

Regarding barium swallow examination of the oesophagus in oesophageal dysmotility disorders, which of the following statements are correct?
(Multiple answers might be correct.)

1. Corkscrew or rosary bead appearance is typical of diffuse oesophageal spasm
2. Achalasia shows a dilated intrathoracic oesophagus
3. In scleroderma, the peristalsis is reduced or absent
4. Tapering of the distal oesophagus towards lower oesophageal sphincter is typical of scleroderma
5. In achalasia, a drink during the exam may help visualise sphincter relaxation and barium emptying

❓ MRQ 7

A 44-year-old patient with chronic renal failure:
- Pain and inflammatory blood work
- Unenhanced CT of the abdomen is performed

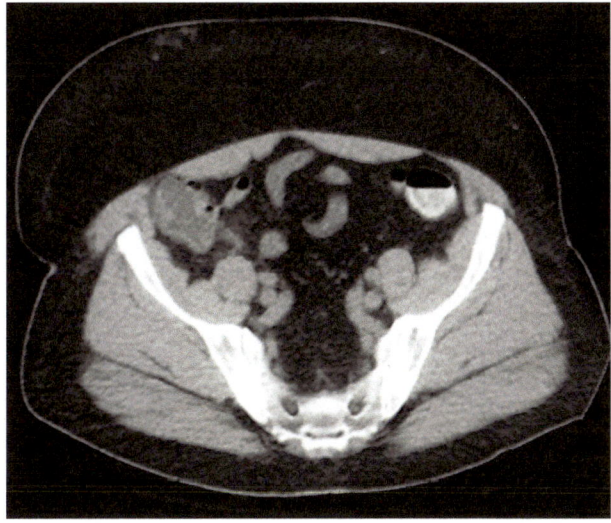

1

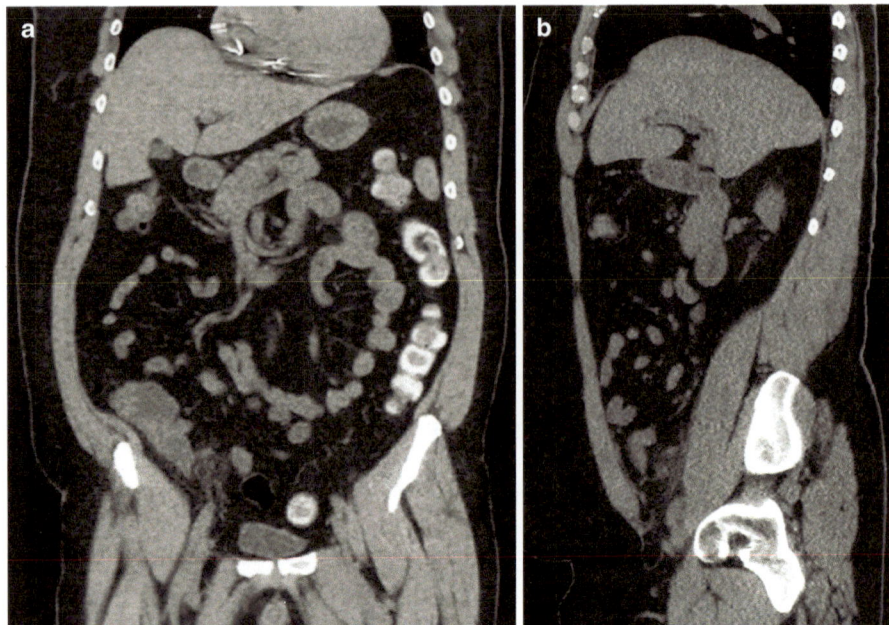

Which of the following statements are true?
(Multiple answers might be correct.)
1. There are inflammatory changes at the ileocoecal region
2. Appendicitis is a likely differential diagnosis
3. Colorectal cancer should also be considered as a differential diagnosis
4. Appendicitis epiploica (epiploic appendagitis) immediately adjacent to the appendix is a likely differential diagnosis
5. Renal insufficiency is known as a trigger for the underlying disease

? **MRQ 8**
Which of the following statements are important for the management of abdominal aortic aneurysms?
(Multiple answers might be correct.)
1. Patient gender
2. Location of the aneurysm
3. Patient age
4. Differentiation between ruptured and non-ruptured
5. Aneurysm size

MRQ 9

Regarding ileus, which of the following statements are true?

(Multiple answers might be correct.)

1. A gallstone may be found inside the intestine
2. Ileus may be caused by arterial or venous ischaemia
3. Previous abdominal surgery is a common association
4. Gas in portal system is one indicator for advanced stages and worsened outcome
5. Volvulus is a rather rare cause

MRQ 10

Regarding the image below:

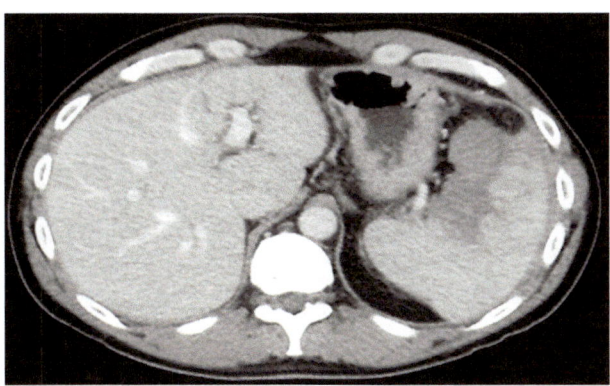

Using the OIS (Organ Injury Scale) by Moore, the splenic injury would be graded as:

(Only one option is correct.)

1. Grade 1: Haematoma subcapsular, non-expanding, <10% surface area, non-bleeding, <1 cm parenchymal depth
2. Grade 2: Haematoma subcapsular, non-expanding, 10–50% surface area, active bleeding, 1–3 cm parenchymal depth
3. Grade 3: Haematoma subcapsular, >50% surface area or expanding, ruptured subcapsular haematoma with active bleeding, laceration >3 cm parenchymal depth
4. Grade 4: Haematoma ruptured, intraparenchymal haematoma with active bleeding, major devascularisation (>25% of spleen)
5. Grade 5: Completely shattered spleen

Short Cases (SCs)

1

SC 1

An 87-year-old female:
— Presented to the emergency department with abdominal pain

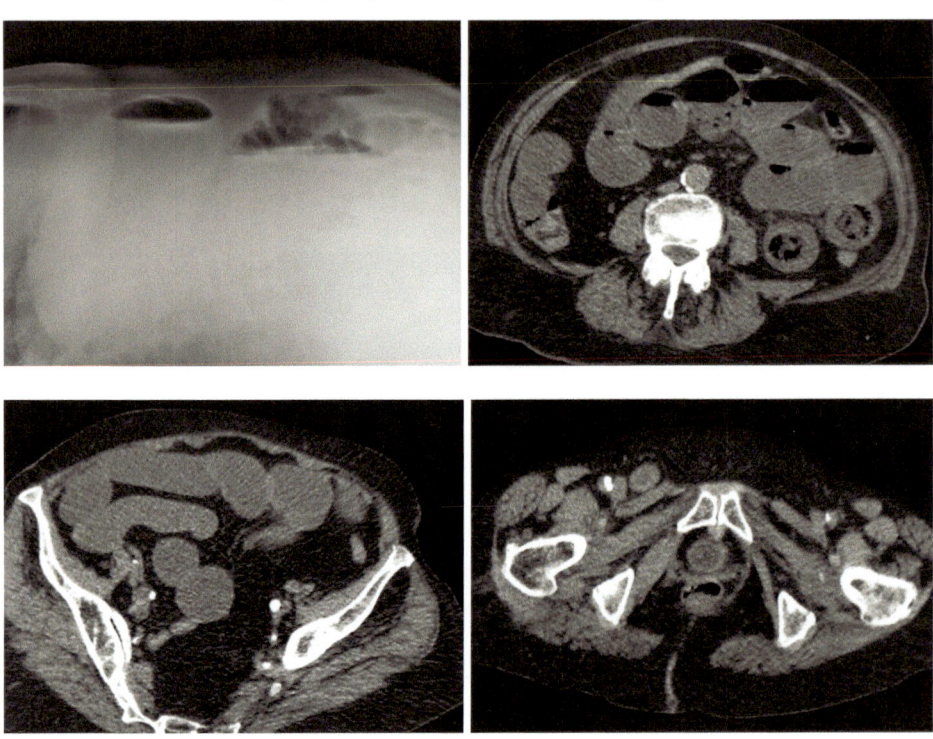

? **Q1**
Indicate the abnormality.

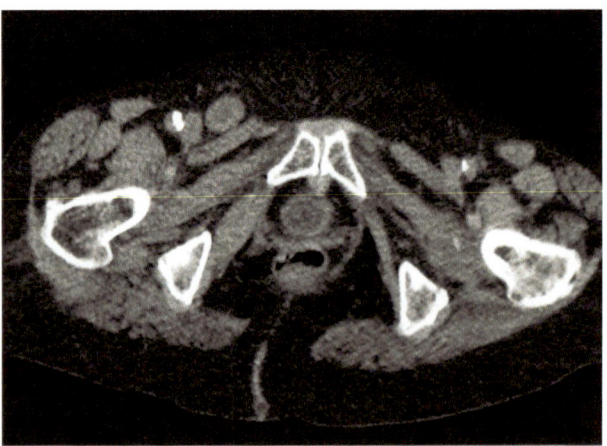

? **Q2**
What is the most likely diagnosis?
(Only one option is correct.)
1. GI bleeding
2. Inflammatory bowel disease
3. Incarcerated right inguinal hernia
4. Large bowel obstruction
5. Small bowel obstruction

? **Q3**
Give the specific cause for the small bowel obstruction shown in this case.

_____

_____

_____

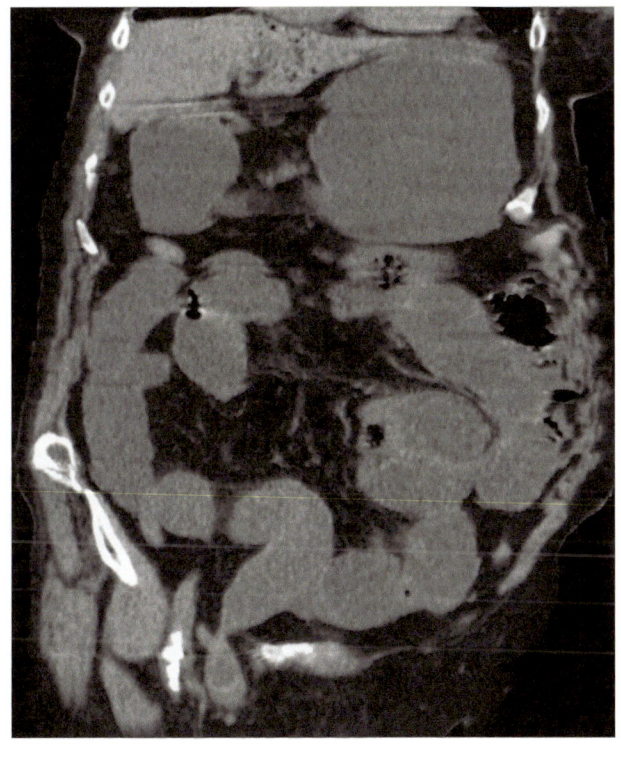

SC 2

1

A 60-year-old male:
- Bright blood per rectum
- No relevant past medical history

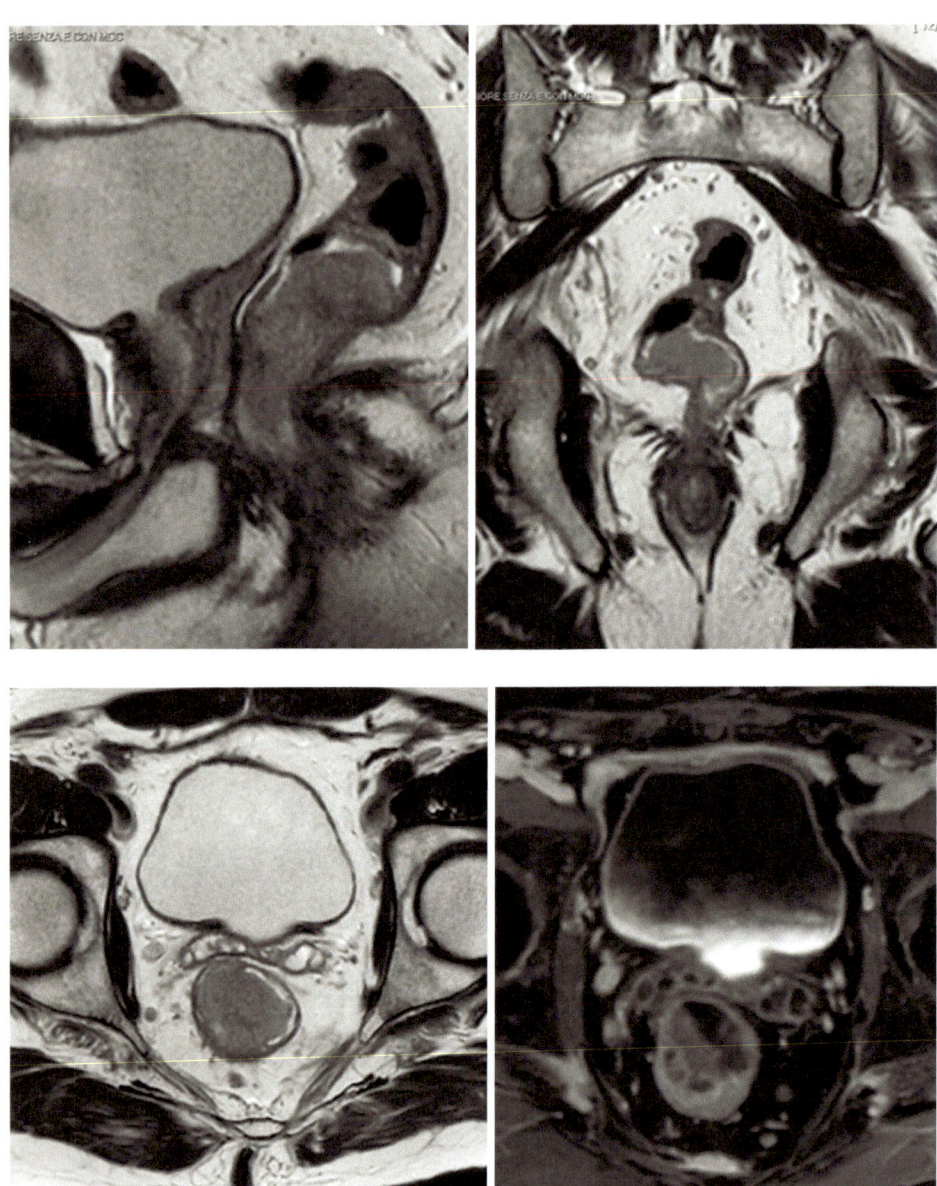

Q1
What radiological features do you recognise in this image?
(Multiple answers might be correct.)
1. Free intraperitoneal fluid
2. Normal/normal variant
3. Mass in the lumen of the rectum
4. Mesorectal nodes
5. Rectal perforation

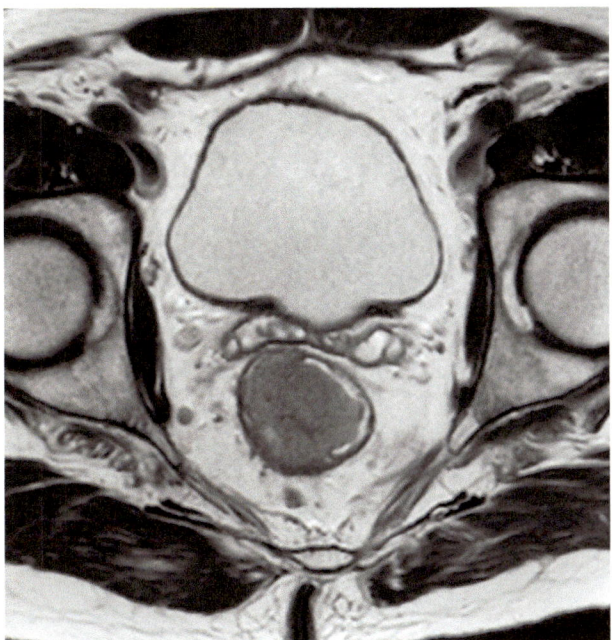

Q2
Differential diagnosis includes:
(Multiple answers might be correct.)
1. Crohn's disease
2. Proctitis
3. Ulcerative colitis
4. Rectal carcinoma
5. Carcinoid tumour

Q3
Give the most likely diagnosis.
(Do not use more than five words.)

❓ Q4
What course of action would you take next?
(Multiple answers might be correct.)
1. Surgical assessment
2. Total body CT for staging
3. FDG-PET
4. Capsule endoscopy
5. Small bowel follow-through

SC 3

A 52-year-old male:
- 5 days following minimal invasive (laparoscopic) appendectomy
- Post-operative rise of CRP and white blood cell count

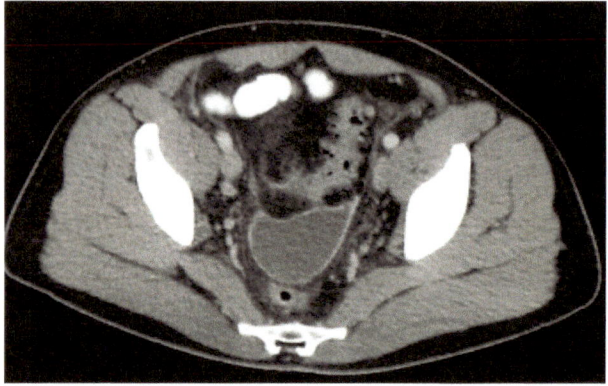

❓ Q1
Indicate the abnormality.

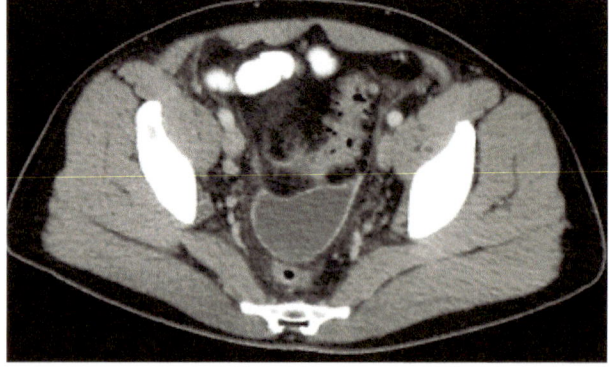

❓ **Q2**
Contrast-enhanced CT was performed in the portal venous phase.

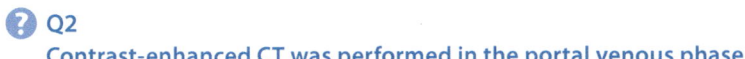

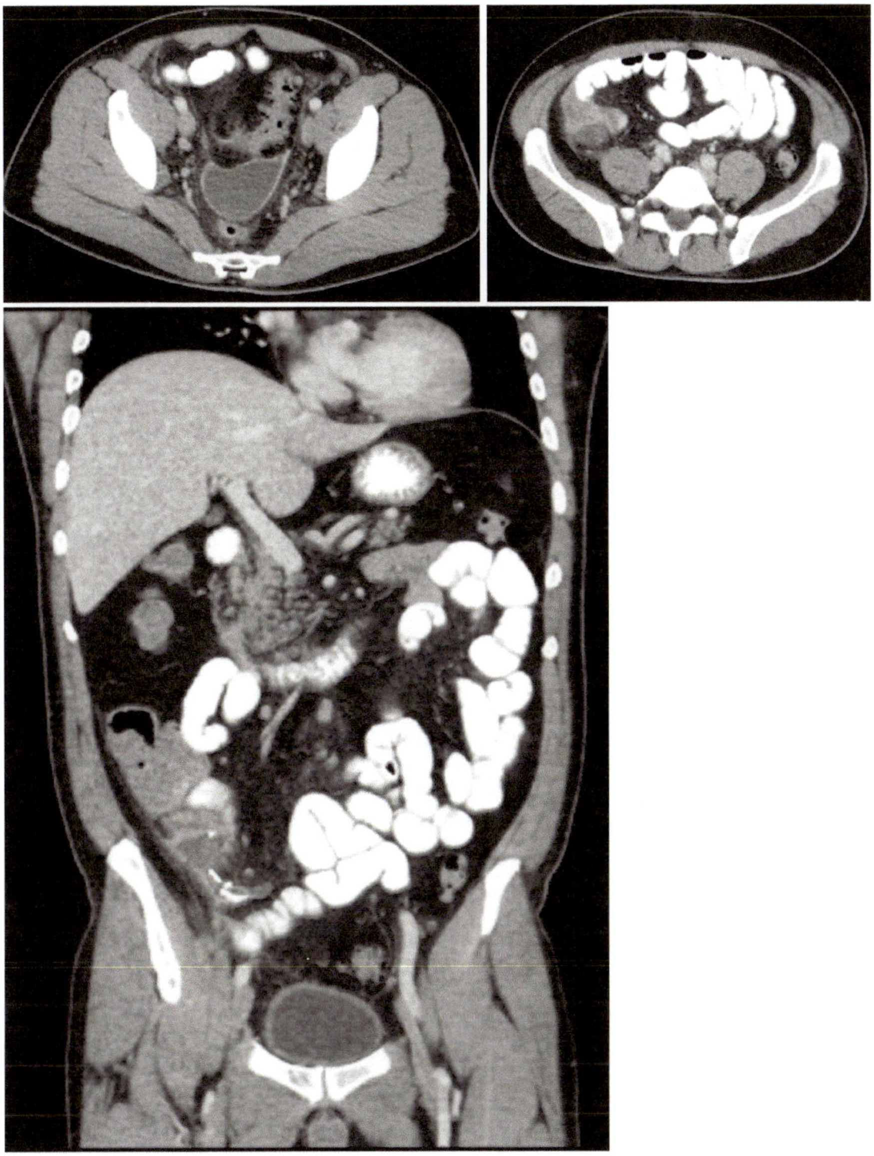

Which of the following findings do you recognise on these images?
(Multiple answers might be correct.)
1. Active bleeding is apparent
2. Ileus is apparent
3. Free abdominal air is apparent
4. Local and mesenteric lymphadenopathy is apparent
5. Swelling of the ileocoecal region is apparent

1

❓ Q3

What is the most likely diagnosis?

(Only one option is correct.)

1. Inflammatory post-operative fluid collection
2. Generalised peritonitis
3. Subphrenic abscess
4. Post-operative perforation of the caecum
5. Ileus in relation with band adhesion

❓ Q4

What course of action would you take next?

(Multiple answers might be correct.)

1. Drain fluid collection
2. Repeat scan with rectal filling
3. Wait and see
4. Embolisation
5. MRI

SC 4

A 66-year-old female:

- Weight loss
- Dysphagia

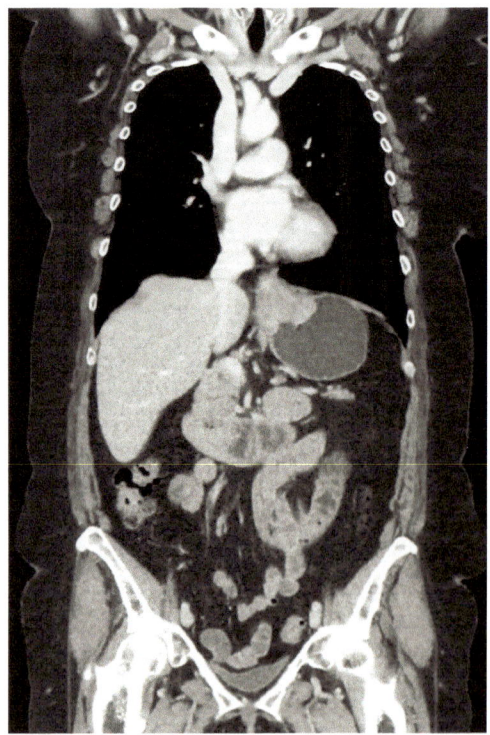

❓ Q1
Indicate the abnormality.

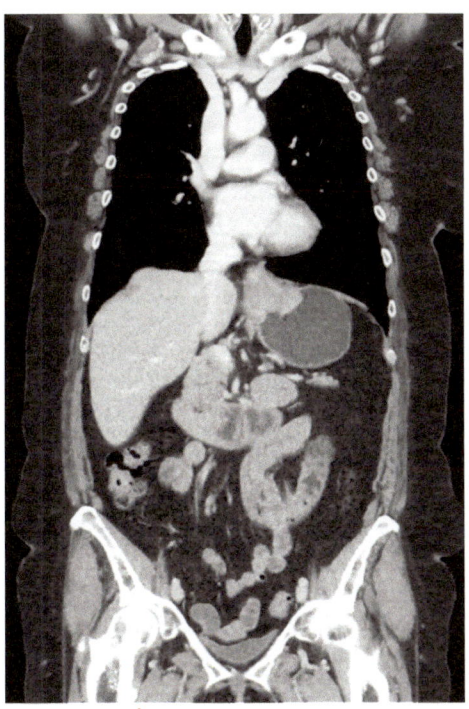

❓ Q2
Where is the lesion located?

_____

_____

_____

1

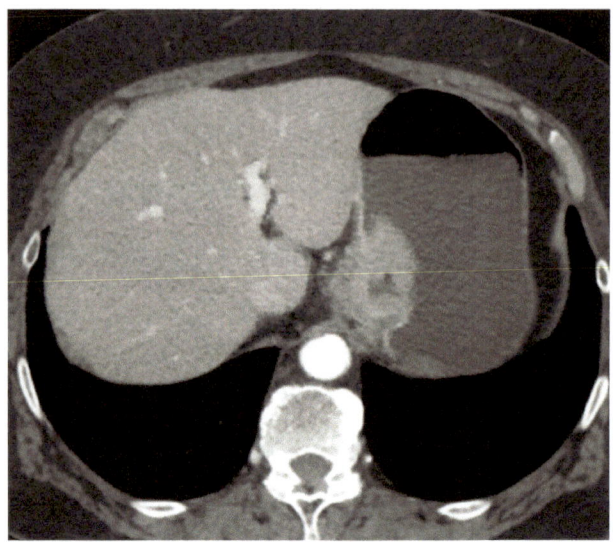

? Q3
Give the most likely diagnosis.

_____

_____

_____

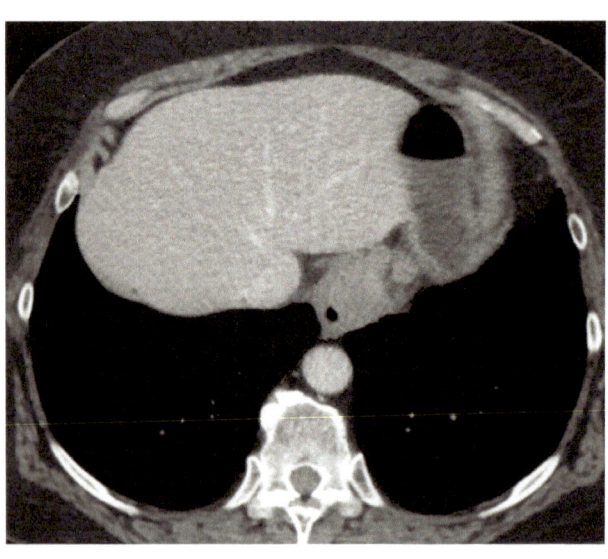

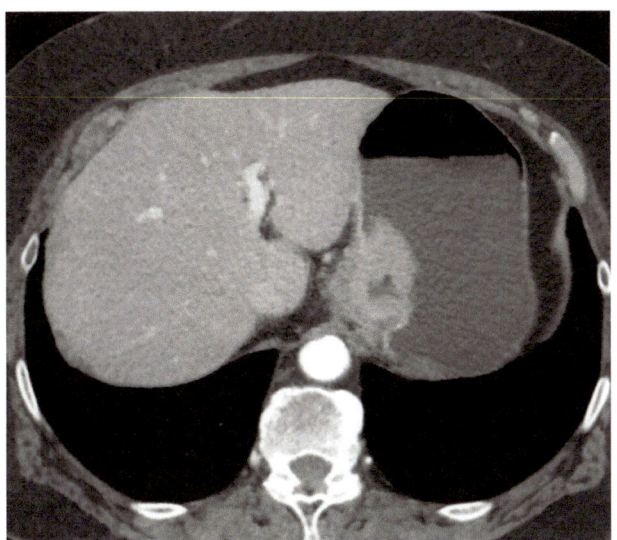

❓ Q4

What are risk factors for development of cancer of the gastroesophageal junction?

(Multiple answers are correct.)

1. Alcohol
2. Tobacco
3. History of pharyngeal cancer
4. Candidiasis
5. Epiphrenic oesophageal diverticulum

❓ Q5

What would you do next for staging?

(Only one option is correct.)

1. MRI of the liver with non-specific gadolinium chelates
2. MRI of the liver with liver-specific MR contrast agent
3. Endosonography
4. Mediastinoscopy
5. Double-contrast upper GI study

CORE

A 70-year-old woman:

— Presenting with abdominal distension and pain

❓ Q1
Describe the key findings.

_____

_____

_____

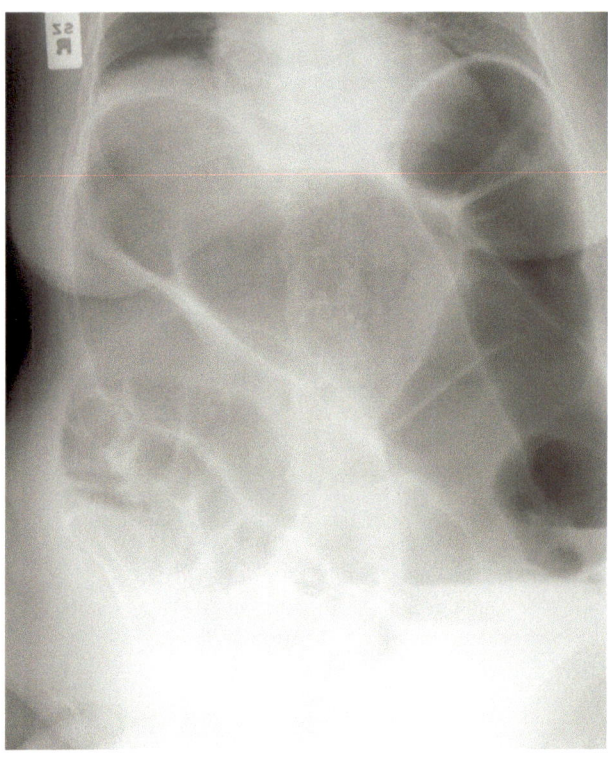

Q2

Describe the key normal and abnormal findings.

Axial CT:

- Video 1.1

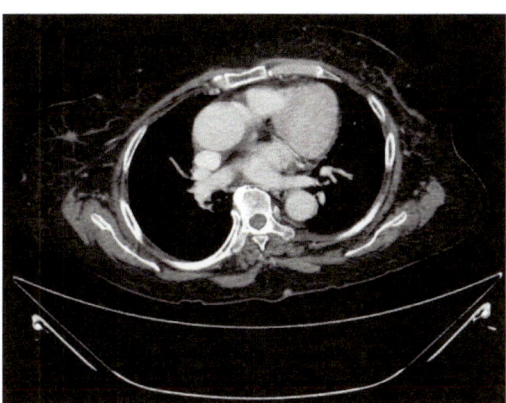

Coronal CT:

- Video 1.2

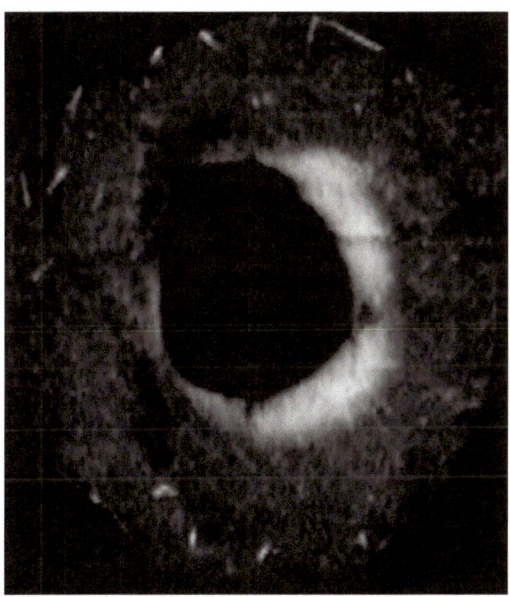

_____

_____

_____

1

? Q3

Please indicate the level of obstruction (zone of transition).

■   **Video 1.3**

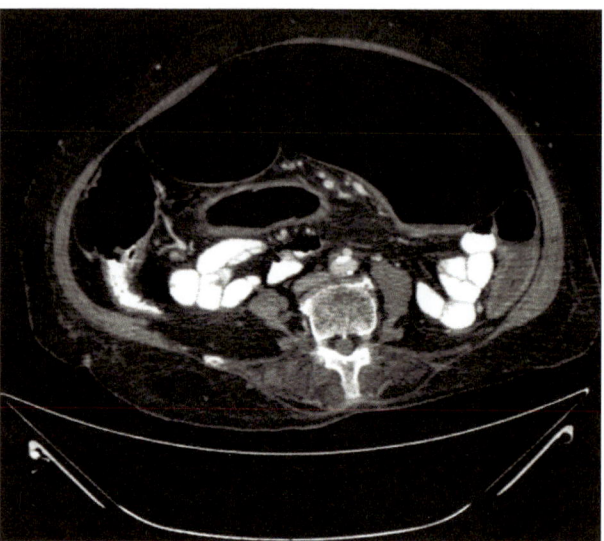

_____

_____

_____

? Q4

What is your diagnosis?

(Only one option is correct.)

1. Intussusception
2. Tumoural obstruction
3. Volvulus
4. Ogilvie syndrome
5. Perforation with adynamic ileus

? Q5

The diagnosis of this patient is sigmoid volvulus. What should be the first attempt for treatment in this patient?

(Only one option is correct.)

1. Laparoscopic detorsion
2. Contrast instillation per rectum
3. Colonoscopic detorsion
4. Percutaneous colonic decompression
5. Laparotomy and surgical treatment

Answers

Multiple Response Questions (MRQs)

 MRQ 1

1

Explanation

The Couinaud classification is the preferred anatomy classification system and divides the liver into eight independent functional units called segments.

    The hepatic veins separate four sections of the liver, each made of two segments on top of each other. The right hepatic vein divides the right lobe into right lateral (posterior) and right medial (anterior) sections. The middle hepatic vein divides the liver into right and left lobes. The left hepatic vein divides the left lobe into left medial and left lateral sections.

    A horizontal plane, running along where the portal vein bifurcates and becomes horizontal, then divides each section of the liver into superior and inferior segments:

- Left lateral section: segment II above and segment III below the portal plane
- Left medial section: segment IVa above and segment IVb below the portal plane
- Right anterior (or medial) section: segment VIII above and segment V below the portal plane
- Right posterior (or lateral) section: segment VII above and segment VI below the portal plane

 MRQ 2

2

Explanation

Schatzki ring is a symptomatically narrow oesophageal B-ring occurring in the distal oesophagus, usually associated with a hiatus hernia.

    Single-contrast solid barium swallows (especially in the RAO prone position) are more sensitive than endoscopy in detecting Schatzki rings.

    A full-column barium swallow will reveal a circumferential narrowing at the gastroesophageal junction, often a few centimetres above the diaphragmatic hiatus, appearing as a thin smooth ring, 1–3 mm thick.

 MRQ 3

2

Explanation

RECIST 1.1 allows selection of up to five target lesions, with a maximum of two lesions per organ. Lesions should be measured in the longest diameter, except for lymph nodes that should be measured in the short axis.

 MRQ 4

3

Explanation

On MR cholangiography, a hilar stricture with dilation of upstream intrahepatic ducts as well as a distal CBD stricture is seen, and multifocal strictures of the main pancreatic duct are also noted.

1

CE-CT and CE-T1WI demonstrate no avid enhancement of the bile duct wall at the stricture site, which is unusual for bile duct cancers, and show a peripancreatic enhancing rim, typical of IgG4-related pancreatitis.

✅ MRQ 5

1 and 3

Explanation

Radiation enteritis affects 5–15% of patients treated with radiotherapy in the abdomen or pelvis. In the acute phase, at Small Bowel Series, the small bowel loops appear spastic, with oedema of the mucosal folds, resulting in luminal narrowing.

✅ MRQ 6

1, 2, and 3

Explanation

At barium swallow, diffuse oesophageal spasm has a characteristic appearance of multiple simultaneous contractions causing a corkscrew appearance with segmentation.

Achalasia is a failure of organised oesophageal peristalsis causing impaired relaxation of the lower oesophageal sphincter, resulting in food stasis and often marked dilatation of the oesophagus, which can be demonstrated at barium swallow.

✅ MRQ 7

1, 2, 3 and 4

Explanation

Colorectal cancer should also be considered as a differential diagnosis, *and* there are inflammatory changes at the ileocoecal region, *and* appendicitis epiploica (epiploic appendagitis) immediately adjacent to the appendix is a likely differential diagnosis, *and* acute appendicitis is a likely differential diagnosis.

Epiploic appendagitis may be the result of spontaneous torsion, ischemia or inflammation of an epiploic appendix of the colon. It may clinically mimic acute appendicitis. Adjacent to an oval, paracaecal fatty mass, representing an infarcted or inflamed appendix epiploica, the caecal wall may (like in this case) show mild local reactive thickening. Epiploic appendagitis is usually managed conservatively. As the CT does not include oral/rectal contrast, caecal cancer may be a differential diagnosis, and of course (although less likely in this case), other inflammatory processes which affect the ileocaecal region, like acute appendicitis, also belong to the group of common alternative causes.

✅ MRQ 8

2, 3, 4 and 5

Explanation

Differentiation between ruptured and non-ruptured *and* aneurysm size *and* patient age *and* location of the aneurysmal are all important factors which impact management of abdominal aortic aneurysms.

The patient's gender is irrelevant in terms of therapy. Ageing often brings an increase in comorbidities, the aneurysm size and especially any interval increase in aneurysm diameter are important factors which impact the decision whether surgical therapy is necessary, and of course, the much more critical finding of rupture in comparison to non-ruptured types should result in an immediate interventional/surgical therapy.

✅ MRQ 9

1, 2, 3, and 4

Explanation

Ileus may be caused by arterial or venous ischaemia, *and* a gallstone may be found inside the lumen of the intestine, *and* previous abdominal surgery is a common association, *and* gas in portal system is one indicator for advanced stages and worsened outcome.

Ileus may be paralytic (post-operative, ischaemic) or obstructive (e.g. adhesions following inflammation or surgery; gallstone ileus by direct inflammatory penetration of a gallstone into the intestinal lumen with impaction in more smaller calibre distal loops; invagination; herniation). Considering ischaemia, the most common causes include arterial embolic disease, thrombotic or invasive venous occlusion and strangulation by volvulus.

✅ MRQ 10

3

Explanation

Grade 3: Haematoma subcapsular, >50% surface area or expanding, ruptured subcapsular haematoma with active bleeding, laceration >3 cm parenchymal depth.

The Moore classification is a grading system developed to classify the activeness of bleeding and extent of devascularisation of splenic injuries. The amount of the organ area/volume involved and the depth of a laceration are additional helpful criteria. In the given case, there is a ruptured subcapsular hematoma with local distribution but also further haematoma surrounding the liver, but no devascularisation above 25% is visible. This suggests Grade 3 injury.

Short Cases (SCs)

SC 1
 Q1

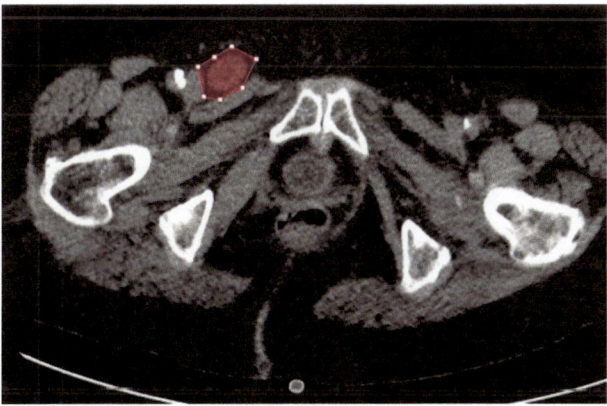

✅ **Q2**

5

✅ **Q3**

Inguinal hernia

Explanation

Supine lateral view CXR and non-contrast-enhanced axial CT show dilated small bowel loops, with air-fluid levels. The fourth image shows a structure in the right inguinal canal, which is suspicious for a herniated bowel loop, confirmed on the coronal image that is subsequently provided. The diagnosis therefore is small bowel obstruction secondary to incarcerated right inguinal hernia.

SC 2

✅ **Q1**

3 and 4

✅ **Q2**

4 and 5

✅ **Q3**

Rectal carcinoma

✅ **Q4**

1, 2 and 3

Explanation

The MRI images show a mass inside the lumen of the rectum, consistent with a neoplasm. In the post-contrast image, the mass is not hypervascular, therefore more compatible with carcinoma than with carcinoid. Small round-shaped nodes are visible in the mesorectum.

SC 3

✅ **Q1**

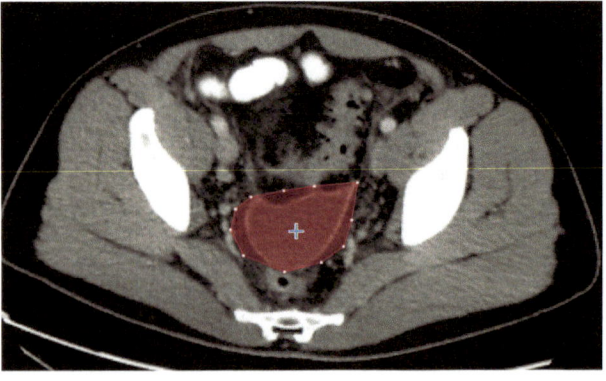

Answers

✓ **Q2**

4 and 5

✓ **Q3**

1

Explanation

Consider clinical data: 5 days following minimal invasive (laparoscopic) appendectomy *and* post-operative rise of CRP and white blood cell count.

   Note: Inflammation in the region of the ileocoecal junction and the ileocaecal
valve (in direct vicinity of surgical clips) and fluid collection in the space of Douglas
with enhancing borders.

✓ **Q4**

1

Explanation

Interventional drainage is a very powerful tool and often results in avoidance of
additional surgical procedures.

   (Other answer options: As there is no differential diagnosis, there is no need for
further imaging. No active bleeding. Wait and see is inappropriate in the given clinical context; at least intravenous antibiotics are required.)

SC 4

✓ **Q1**

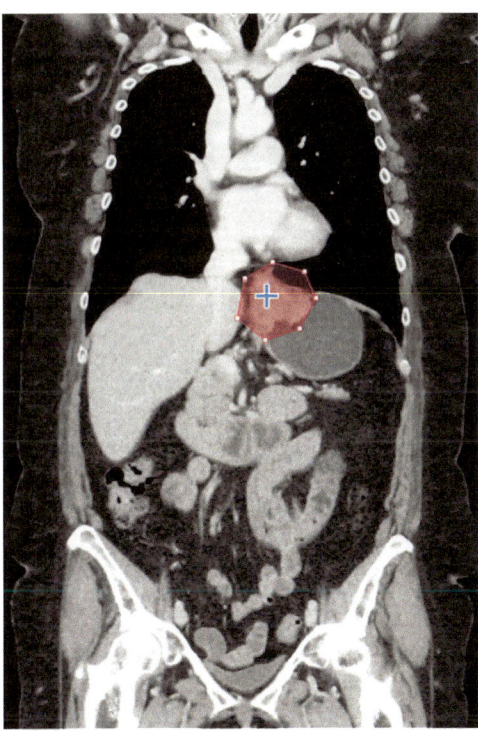

1

✅ **Q2**
Gastroesophageal junction

✅ **Q3**
Cancer

✅ **Q4**
1, 2 and 3

✅ **Q5**
3

CORE

✅ **Q1**
- Distension and dilatation of large bowel loops
- No free air
  Explanation
  Plain abdominal radiograph shows a prominent, dilated loop of colon, which originates in the pelvis, with a fluid level at its lower end. The dilated loop of bowel has few haustrations and extends into the upper abdomen, and its lower end points towards the pelvis. There is no evidence of pneumoperitoneum.

✅ **Q2**

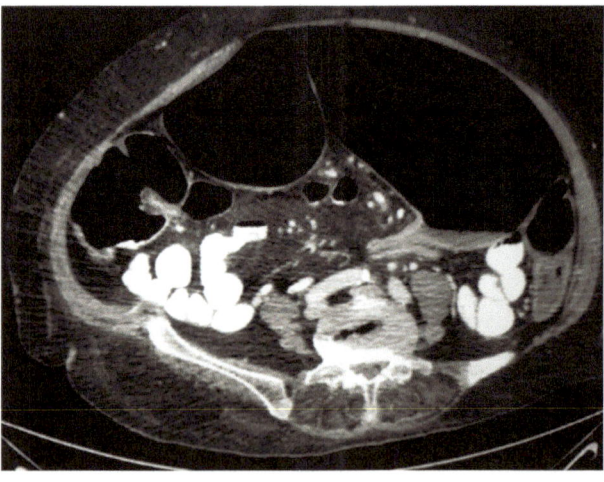

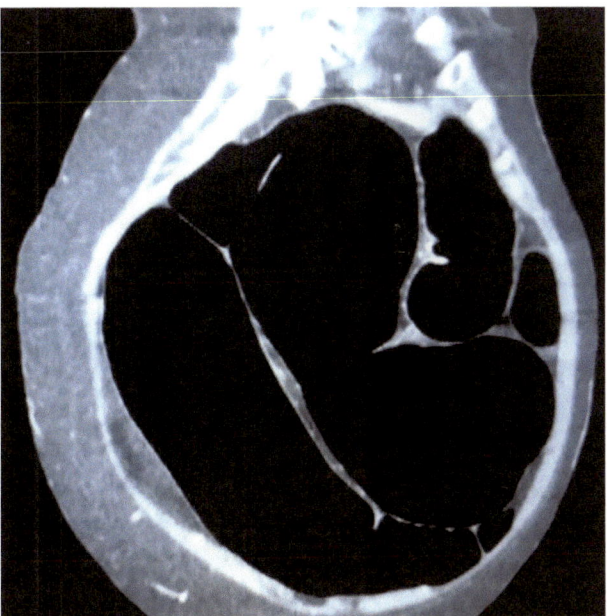

- Distension/dilatation of large bowel down to the sigmoid colon
- Transition zone is at the sigmoid colon
- Twisting of sigmoid mesocolon ("beak sign") at the level of pelvic brim
- Ascites (perihepatic, small volume)
- Gallstones
- Small bowel is not dilated
- No pneumoperitoneum

Explanation

Computed tomography (following intravenous and oral contrast) shows a large, redundant, gas-filled loop of large bowel, lacking haustrations, which originates in the pelvis and extends into the right upper quadrant. At its point of origin at the left pelvic brim, there is a twist of the redundant sigmoid colon on its own mesentery leading to a "whirl sign" with twisting of the mesentery and mesenteric vessels. The loop of dilated sigmoid colon forms a closed loop obstruction, and its appearance is similar to a coffee bean (the "coffee bean" sign).

The small bowel is not dilated. There is no pneumoperitoneum. There is a small volume of perihepatic free fluid.

Incidental cortical loss at the lower pole of the left kidney, likely reflecting chronic pyelonephritic change. There are gallstones in the gallbladder.

✅ Q3

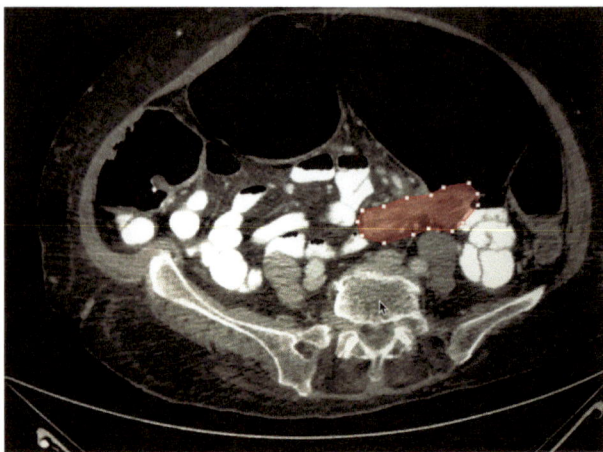

Explanation

At the point of origin of the dilated loop of sigmoid colon at the left pelvic brim, there is a twist of the redundant sigmoid colon on its own mesentery leading to a "whirl sign" with twisting of the mesentery and mesenteric vessels. The site of the twist and "whirl sign" is indicated in red.

✅ Q4
3

✅ Q5
3

Literature

Ciaravino V, De Robertis R, Tinazzi Martini P, et al. Imaging presentation of pancreatic neuroendocrine neoplasms. Insights Imaging. 2018;9(6):943–53.

Eisenhauer EA, Therasse P, Bogaerts J, et al. New response evaluation criteria in solid tumours: Revised RECIST guideline (version 1.1). Eur J Cancer. 2009;45(2):228–47.

Florim S, Almeida A, Rocha D, Portugal P. Acute mesenteric ischaemia: a pictorial review. Insights Imaging. 2018;9(5):673–82.

Lee NK, Kim S, Jeon TY, et al. Complications of Congenital and Developmental Abnormalities of the Gastrointestinal Tract in Adolescents and Adults: Evaluation with Multimodality Imaging. Radiographics. 2010;30:1489–507.

Onur MR, Akpinar E, Karaosmanoglu AD, Isayev C, Karcaaltincaba M. Diverticulitis: a comprehensive review with usual and unusual complications. Insights Imaging. 2017;8(1):19–27.

Salati U, McNeill G, Torreggiani WC. The coffee bean sign in sigmoid volvulus. Radiology. 2011;258: 651–2.

Tirkes T, Hollar MA, Tann M, Kohli MD, Akisik F, Sandrasegaran K. Response criteria in oncologic imaging: review of traditional and new criteria. Radiographics. 2013;33(5):1323–41.

Vilaça AF, Reis AM, Vidal IM. The anatomical compartments and their connections as demonstrated by ectopic air. Insights Imaging. 2013;4:759–72.

Additional EDiR Preparatory Materials

http://learn.myesr.org

EDiR Preparatory Sessions

http://learn.myesr.org
Imaging of the most frequent emergencies of the GI tract.
Benign hepatocellular tumours: how to differentiate.
Imaging of cystic masses of the pancreas.

Breast Radiology

© European Board of Radiology (EBR) 2019
J. Babar et al., *EDiR - The Essential Guide*, https://doi.org/10.1007/978-3-030-20066-4_2

Multiple Response Questions (MRQs)

2

❓ MRQ 1

A 52-year-old symptomatic woman. Breast US is performed.

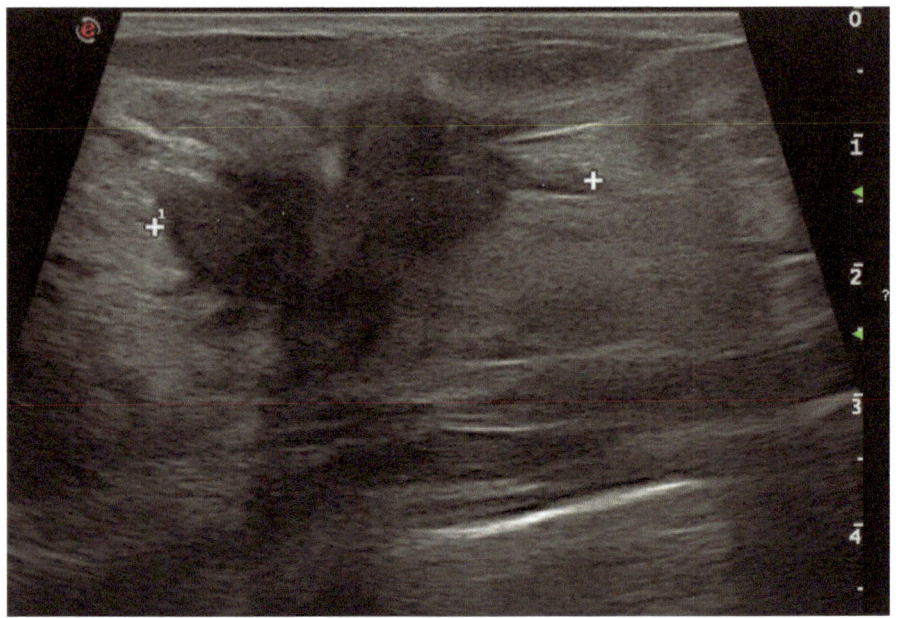

Which of the following statements are correct regarding this image?
(Multiple answers might be correct.)

1. The most likely diagnosis is invasive carcinoma
2. This lesion is highly suggestive of malignancy
3. This lesion is probably benign
4. The most likely diagnosis is ductal carcinoma in situ
5. An additional core needle biopsy is necessary

MRQ 2
Magnified paddle view of a lesion in the left breast:

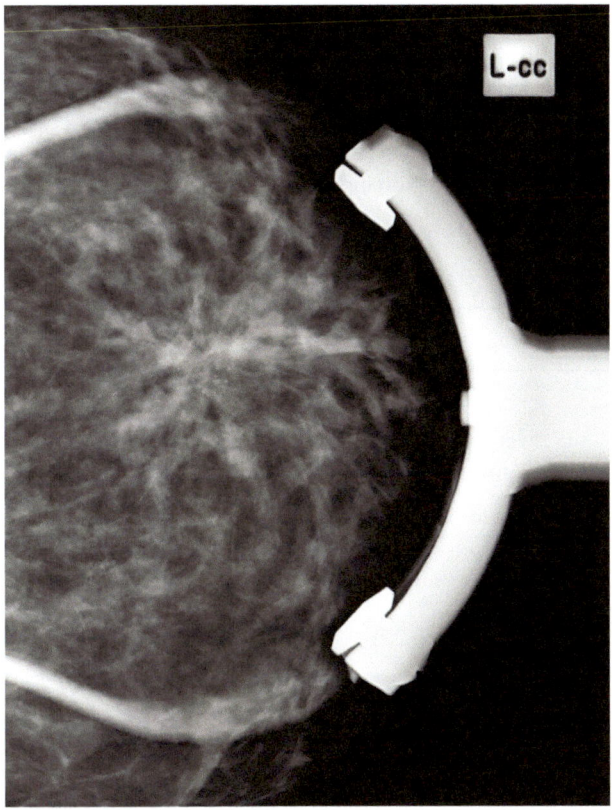

Differential diagnosis includes:
(Multiple answers might be correct.)
1. Radial scar
2. Invasive carcinoma
3. Fat necrosis
4. Post-operative changes
5. Fibroadenoma

MRQ 3
Which of the following statements regarding stereotactic guided breast biopsy are correct?
(Multiple answers might be correct.)
1. It is usually performed without local anaesthesia
2. It is the method of choice for the assessment of suspicious microcalcifications
3. No ionising radiation is used
4. It is preferentially used with a vacuum-assisted large-core needle biopsy device
5. It is performed with the patient in supine position

2

❓ **MRQ 4**

Regarding the evaluation of breast implants, which of the following statements are correct?

(Multiple answers might be correct.)

1. MRI has a higher sensitivity for detecting implant rupture than ultrasound
2. The linguine sign is a reliable indicator for intracapsular implant rupture with breast MRI
3. MRI can differentiate intracapsular from extracapsular implant rupture
4. Expanders can be safely evaluated with breast MRI without significant artefacts
5. Radial folds seen on breast MRI is a strong indicator of implant rupture

Short Cases (SCs)

SC 1

A 55-year-old patient:

– Bilateral cosmetic implants inserted 10 years ago

– Presents with a smooth mobile lump in the upper outer quadrant of the left breast

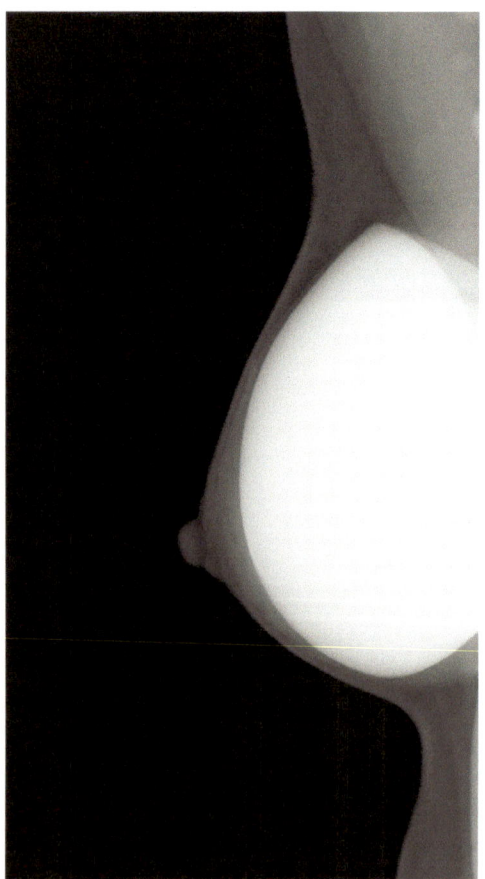

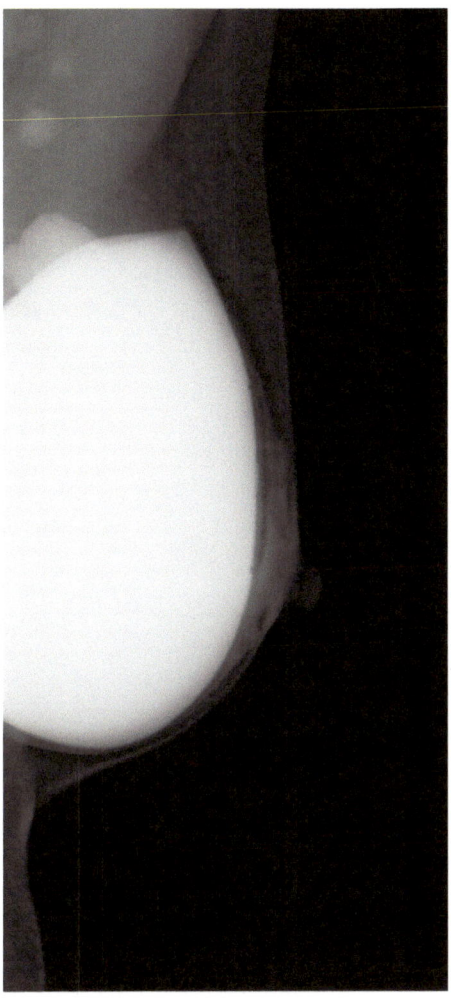

🔲 Bilateral MLO mammograms

❷ Q1
Indicate the abnormality.

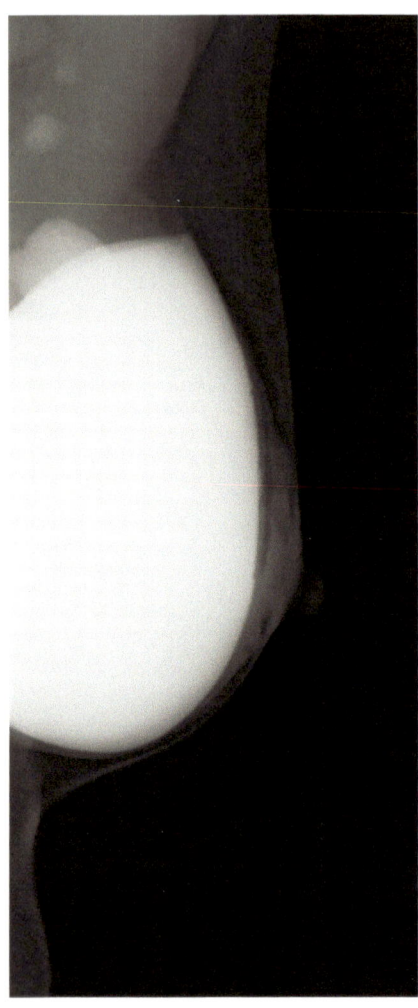

❓ Q2
Breast ultrasound is performed.

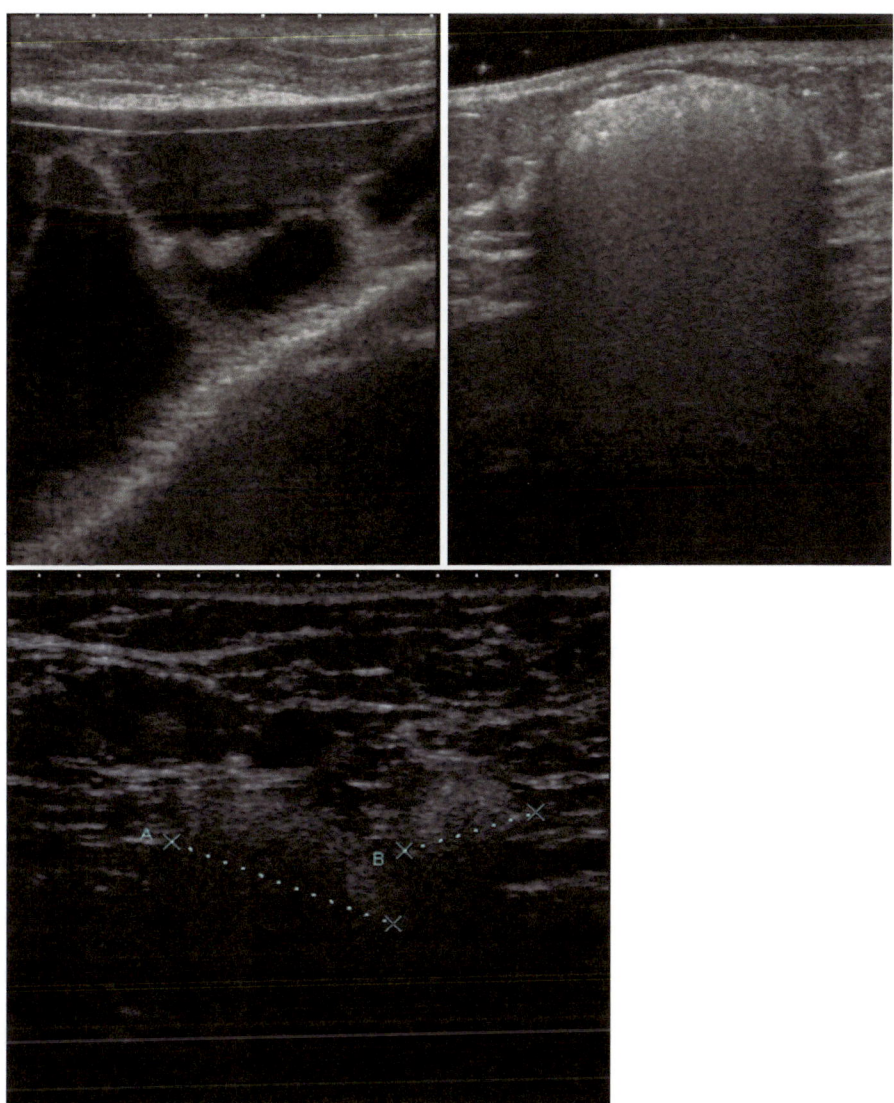

What BIRADS classification would you give to this ultrasound?
(Only one option is correct.)
1. Normal (BIRADS 1)
2. Benign (BIRADS 2)
3. Suspicious probably benign (BIRADS 3)
4. Suspicious probably malignant (BIRADS 4)
5. Malignant (BIRADS 5)

2

❓ Q3

What is the most likely diagnosis?

(Only one option is correct.)

1. Intracapsular implant rupture and silicone in lymph nodes
2. Extracapsular implant rupture and silicone in lymph nodes
3. Intracapsular implant rupture and reactive lymph nodes
4. Intracapsular and extracapsular implant rupture and reactive lymph node
5. Intracapsular and extracapsular implant rupture and silicone in lymph nodes

SC 2

A 56-year-old woman:

— Presented with left breast discomfort and nodularity in the upper outer quadrant of the left breast, which is clinically benign

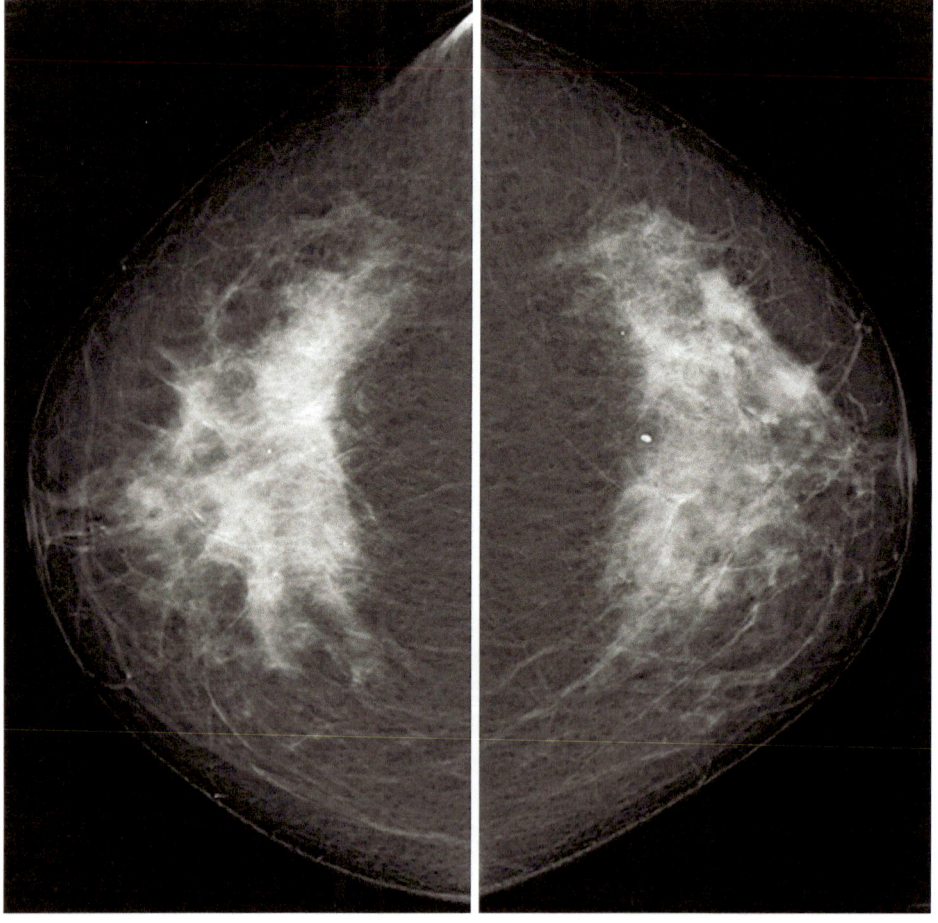

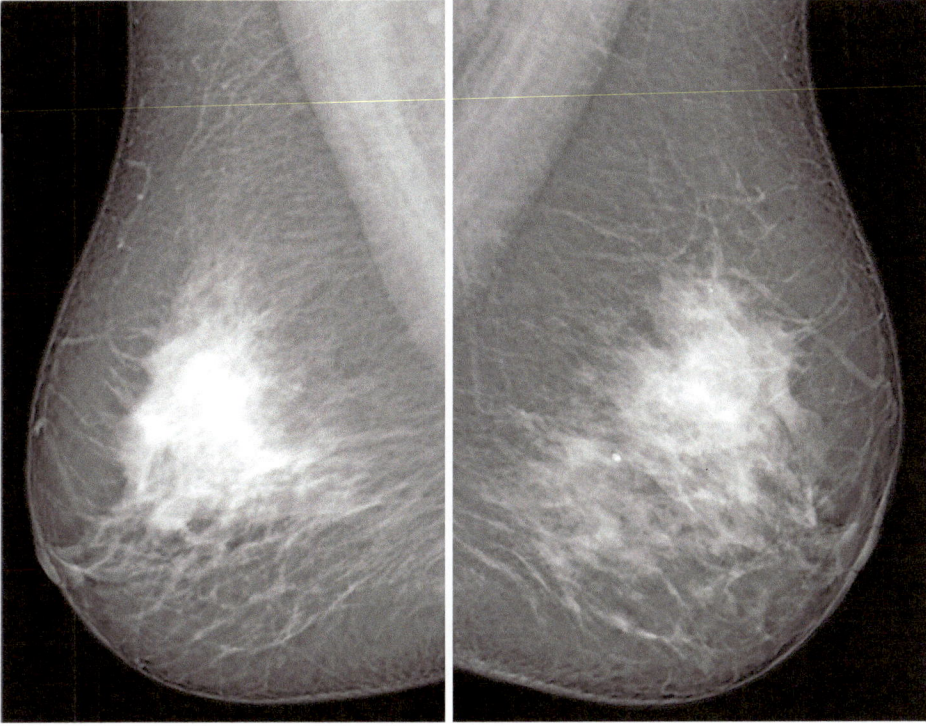

❓ Q1

How would you report these mammograms?

(Multiple answers might be correct.)

1. There are scattered areas of fibroglandular density (breast composition "b")
2. The breasts are heterogeneously dense (breast composition "c")
3. As it is clinically benign, follow-up in 3–6 months is required
4. Further imaging is needed to assess the left breast
5. Compare them with the previous films if available

2

❓ Q2

Indicate the abnormality.

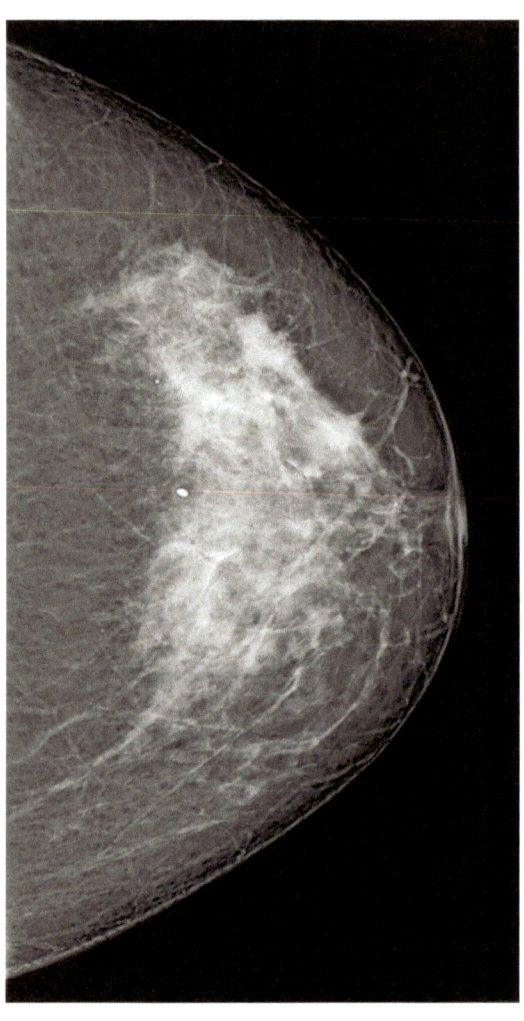

? **Q3**

 — No previous films were available
 — Tomosynthesis was performed to further assess the left breast
Indicate the area of abnormality in this tomosynthesis image

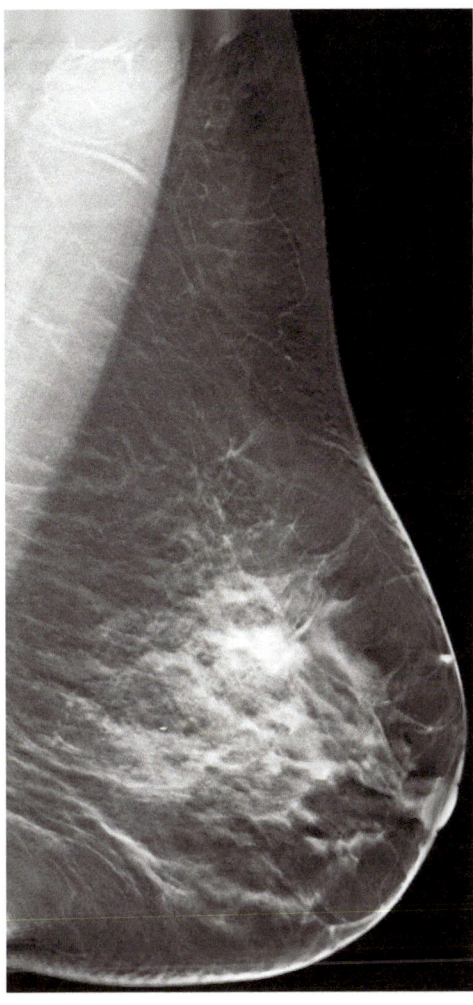

2

 Q4

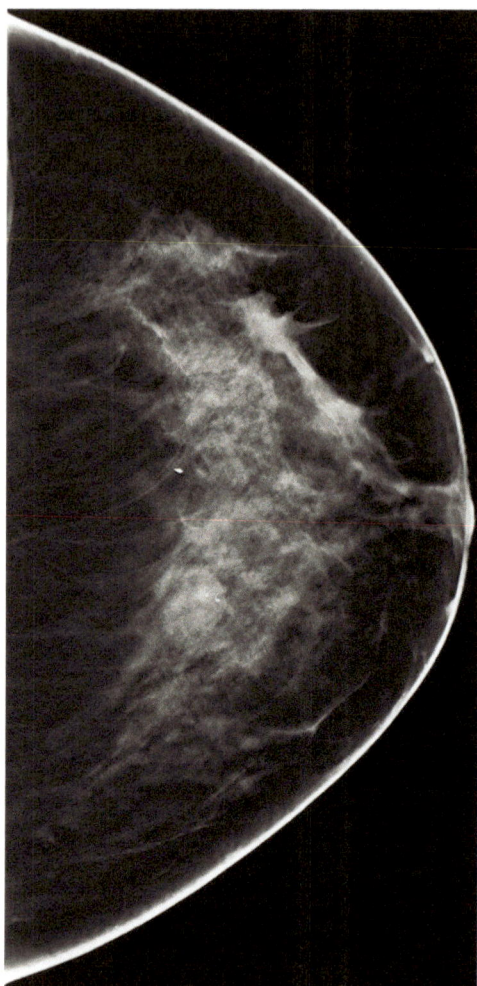

Regarding breast tomosynthesis, which of the following statements are correct?
(Multiple answers might be correct.)
1. There is improved resolution of distortions and masses compared to 2D mammography in all breast
2. The radiation dose is 1.5 times the conventional film-screen 2D mammography
3. Calcifications can be less sharply delineated on tomosynthesis, and therefore 2D magnification views are advised
4. Tomosynthesis can reduce recall rates in breast cancer screening
5. Tomosynthesis has been shown to improve both sensitivity and specificity of cancer detection rates

❓ Q5

Ultrasound examination of the left breast identified an irregular hypoechoic mass in the left breast. It was biopsied under ultrasound guidance.

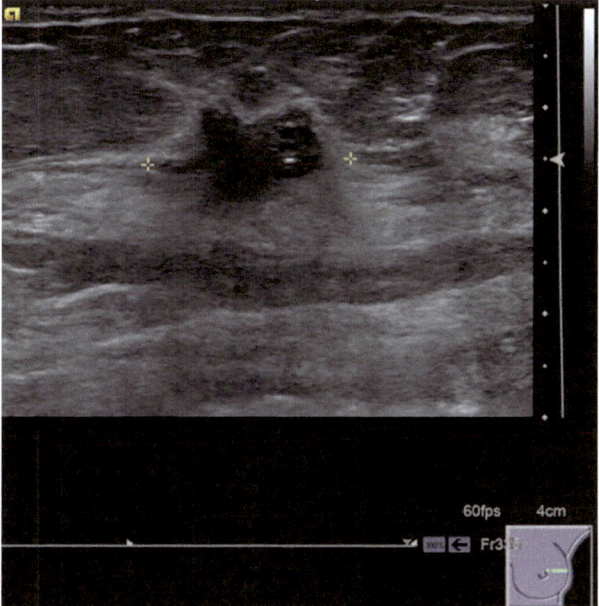

Give the most likely diagnosis:

_____

_____

_____

CORE

A 42-year-old female:
- Palpable mass in the left breast at 3 o'clock position

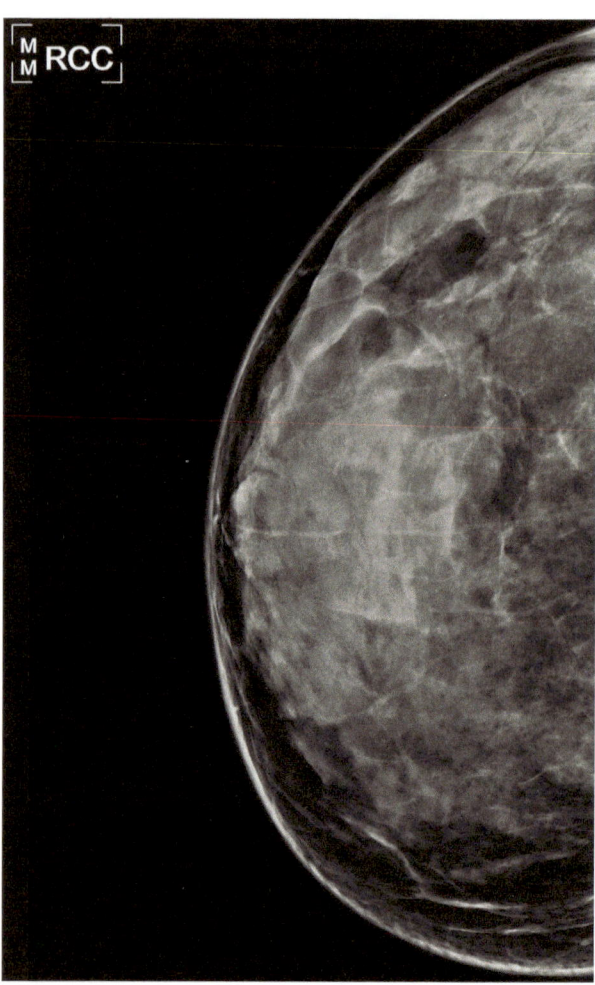

◘ RCC mammography

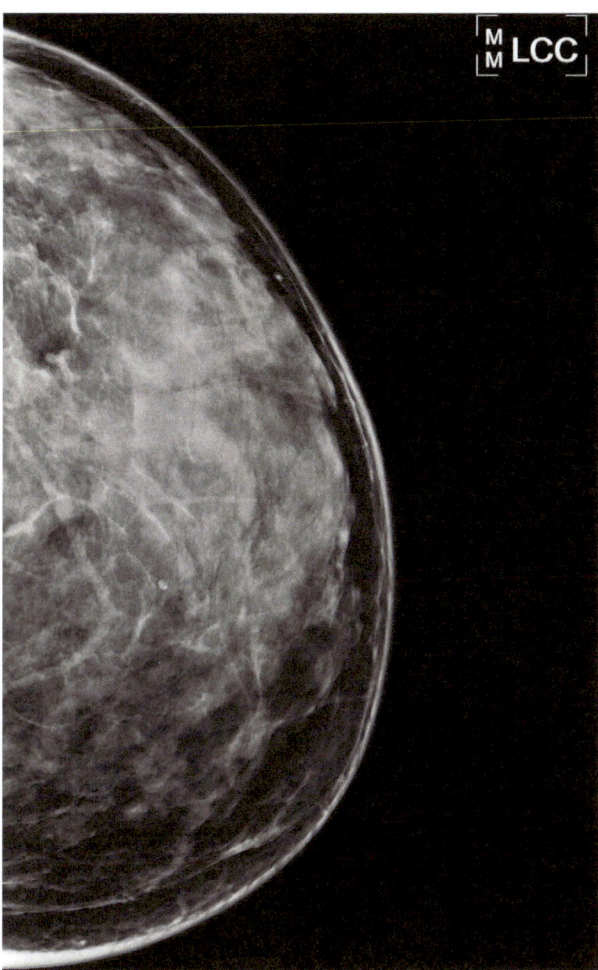

■ LCC mammography

2

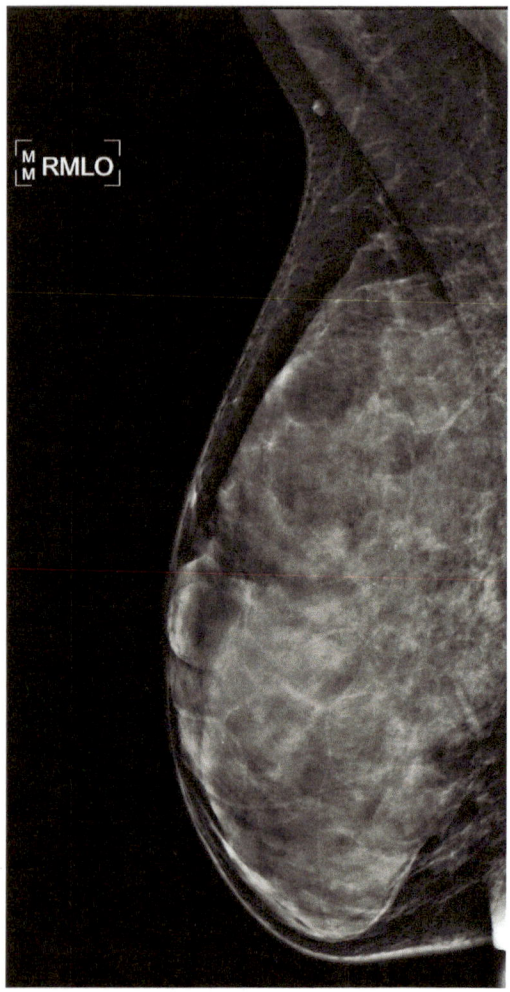

◼ RMLO

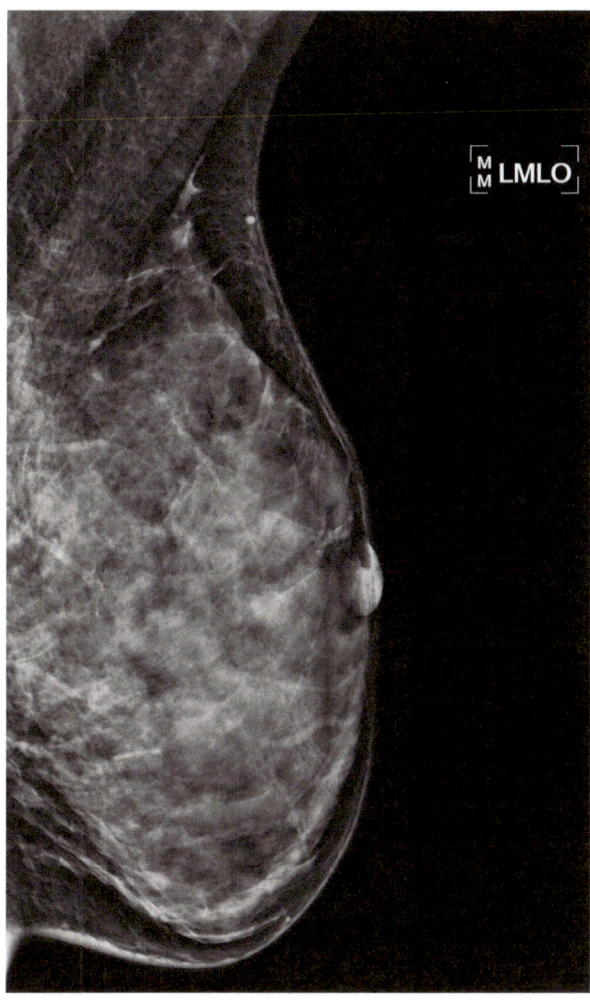

■ LMLO

2

❓ Q1

Describe the mammography findings and advise about the appropriate next step.

_____

_____

_____

❓ Q2
US is performed.

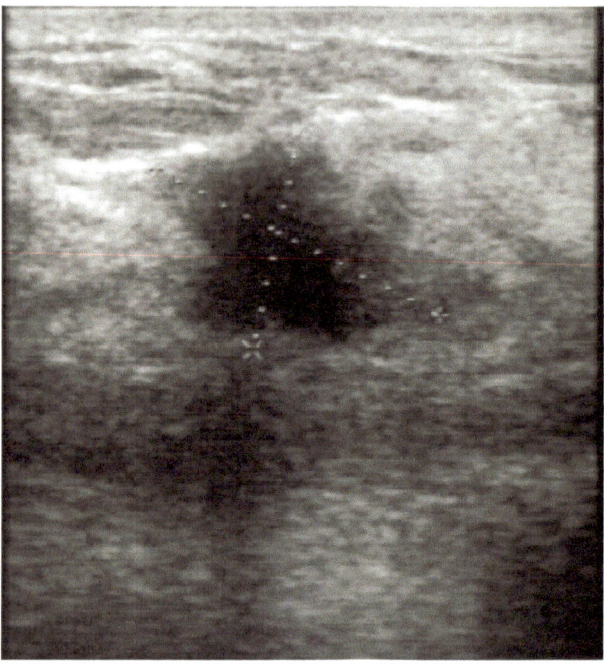

Describe the abnormality.

_____

_____

_____

? **Q3**
How would you grade it according to BIRADS?

_____

_____

_____

? **Q4**
Which is the most likely diagnosis?
(Only one option is correct.)
1. Adenosis tumour
2. Breast cancer
3. Hamartoma
4. Fibrocystic disease lesion
5. Fibroadenoma

Answers

Multiple Response Questions (MRQs)

✔ **MRQ 1**
1, 2 and 5

✔ **MRQ 2**
1 and 2

✔ **MRQ 3**
2 and 4

✔ **MRQ 4**
1, 2 and 3

Short Cases (SCs)

SC 1

2 ✅ Q1

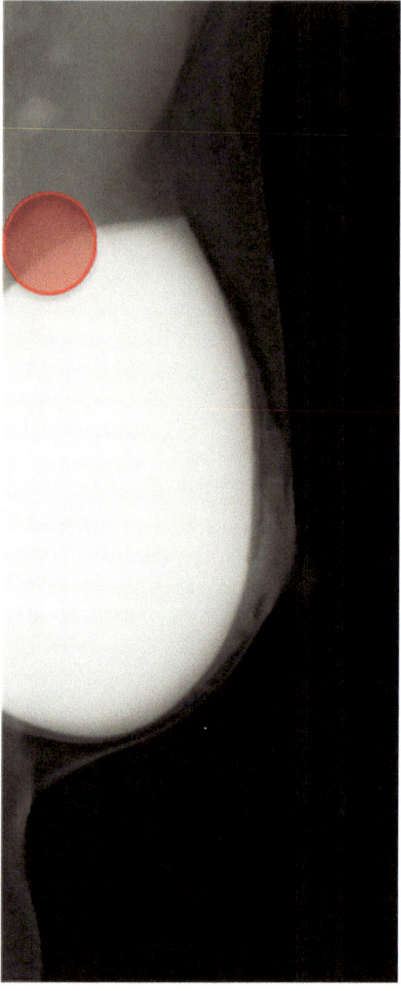

✅ **Q2**

2

✅ **Q3**

5

Explanation

After breast implant surgery, a fibrous capsule forms around the implant shell. Ruptures of breast implants may be intracapsular (more common) whereby the shell of the implant ruptures but the fibrous capsule remains intact, or extracapsular rupture, whereby the fibrous capsule is no longer intact. US sensitivity and specificity of implant rupture is high, although MRI is the most sensitive method of detection of implant rupture. On ultrasound, a stepladder sign of the implant may be seen in intracapsular rupture, with multiple linear internal echoes. A normal implant should be anechoic. A "snowstorm" appearance can be seen in silicone granulomas and silicone containing lymph nodes, which often implies extracapsular rupture.

SC 2

 Q1

2, 4, and 5

 Q2

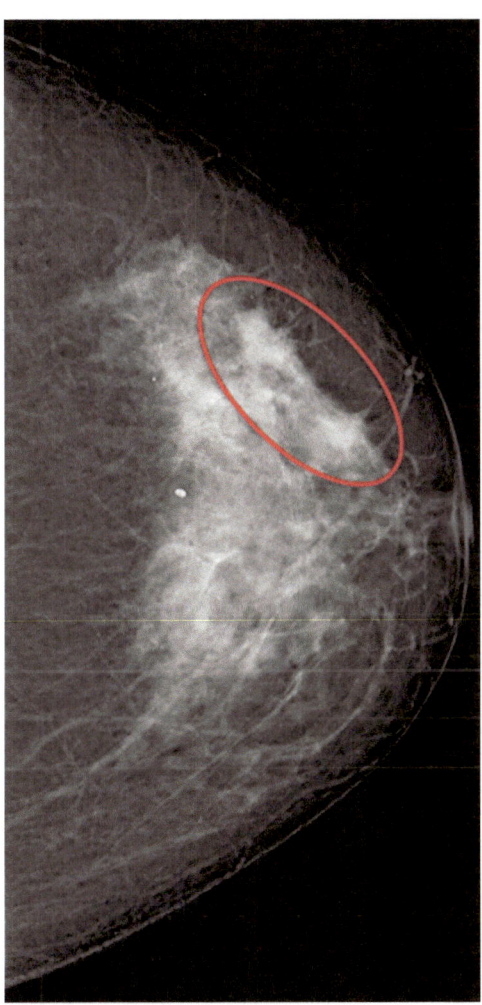

✅ **Q3**

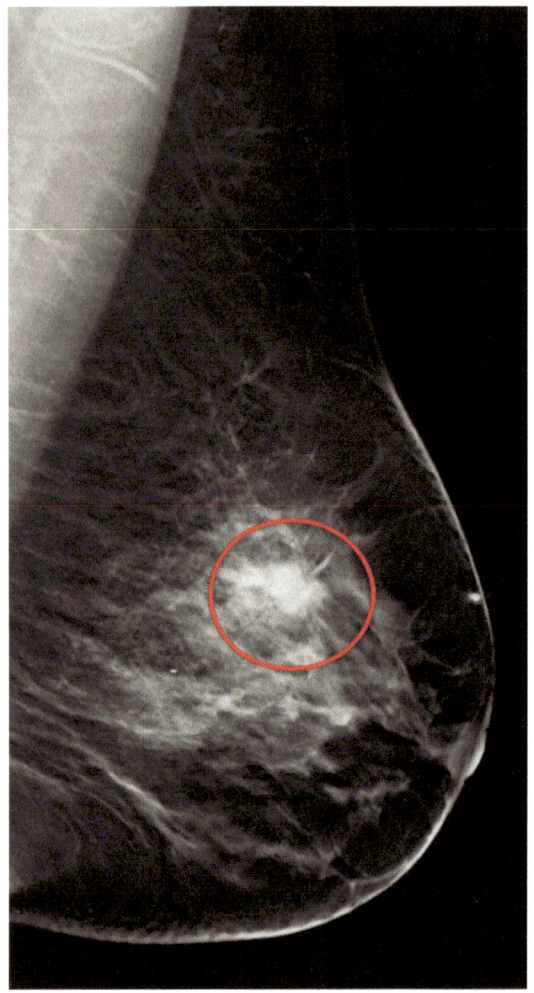

✅ **Q4**
1, 3, 4 and 5

✅ **Q5**
Invasive (ductal or lobular) carcinoma of the breast

CORE

 Q1
- Normal skin and nipple
- Bilateral dense breast tissue
- No microcalcifications
- No suspicious opacity
- Because of the low sensitivity of dense breasts on mammography, additional US should be performed

Q2
- Hypoechoic mass lesion (no through transmission)
- Microlobulated
- Irregular margins

Q3
BIRADS 4b

Q4
2
Explanation
Dense breasts convey an increased risk of malignancy, both due to a masking effect and as an independent risk factor for breast cancer. In women presenting with a palpable lump, US should be performed even if mammography is normal in women with dense breasts. US features of a hypoechoic mass with irregular lobulated margins are highly suspicious for malignancy.

Literature

Dialani V, James DF, Slanetz PJ. A practical approach to imaging the axilla. Insights Imaging. 2015;6(2):217–29.

Dibble EH, Lourenco AP, Baird GL, Ward RC, Maynard AS, Mainiero MB. Comparison of digital mammography and digital breast tomosynthesis in the detection of architectural distortion. Eur Radiol. 2018;28:3.

Joshi S, Dialani V, Marotti J, Mehta TS, Slanetz PJ. Breast disease in the pregnant and lactating patient: radiological-pathological correlation. Insights Imaging. 2013;4(5):527–38.

Juanpere S, Perez E, Huc O, Motos N, Pont J, Pedraza S. Imaging of breast implants—a pictorial review. Insights Imaging. 2011;2(6):653–70.

Mann RM, Kuhl CK, Kinkel K, Boetes C. Breast MRI: guidelines from the European Society of Breast Imaging. Eur Radiol. 2008;18(7):1307–18.

Oliveira TM, Elias J Jr, Melo AF, Teixeira SR, Filho SC, Gonçalves LM, Faria FM, et al. Evolving concepts in breast lobular neoplasia and invasive lobular carcinoma, and their impact on imaging methods. Insights Imaging. 2014;5(2):183–94.

Veltman J, Mann R, Kok T, Obdeijn IM, Hoogerbrugge N, Blickman JG, Boetes C. Breast tumor characteristics of BRCA1 and BRCA2 gene mutation carriers on MRI. Eur Radiol. 2008;18:931.

2

Additional EDiR Preparatory Materials

http://learn.myesr.org

EDiR Preparatory Sessions

http://learn.myesr.org
2D and 3D (tomosynthesis) mammography.
Imaging-guided minimally invasive therapy and breast biopsies.
Clinical challenges on breast MRI.

Cardiac Radiology

Electronic supplementary material The online version of this chapter
(https://doi.org/10.1007/978-3-030-20066-4_3) contains supplementary material,
which is available to authorized users.

Multiple Response Questions (MRQs)

3

❓ MRQ 1

Regarding coronary arteries, which of the following statements are correct?
(Multiple answers might be correct.)
1. The so-called malignant coronary anomalies are more frequent than benign ones
2. Most coronary anomalies are clinically silent
3. ALCAPA (formerly: Bland–White–Garland syndrome) describes a rare coronary anomaly with origin of the left main stem artery from the pulmonary artery
4. Coronary fistulas are not classified as coronary anomalies
5. A retroaortic course of a coronary artery with anomalous origin is named as "malignant coronary anomaly"

❓ MRQ 2

A patient with stable angina, without other risk factors, is referred for noninvasive imaging. Which of the following group of patients with typical angina has a pretest probability of disease for coronary artery disease (CAD) of <66% and is thus considered appropriate?
(Multiple answers might be correct.)
1. Females between 50 and 59 years of age
2. Females younger than 40 years of age
3. Males younger than 40 years of age
4. Males over 60 years of age
5. Females over 65 years of age

❓ MRQ 3

A 48-year-old female patient with sudden onset of chest pain and shortness of breath:

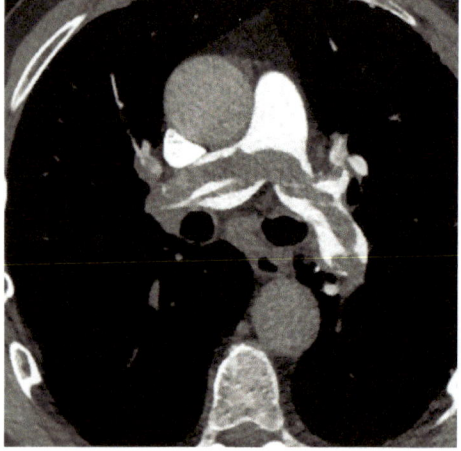 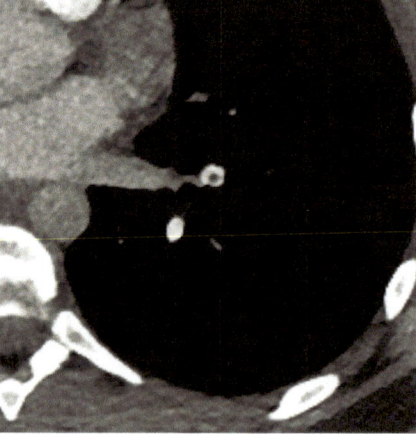

Which of the following statements are correct?
(Multiple answers might be correct.)
1. A negative CT pulmonary angiography should be followed by a ventilation/perfusion (V/Q) scintigraphy
2. MR imaging may be performed as an alternative method in patients who cannot undergo contrast-enhanced CT
3. Acute pulmonary embolism shows a filling defect in the pulmonary artery
4. Subsegmental pulmonary embolism is considered not to be clinically significant
5. Saddle emboli may be seen extending centrally to both the pulmonary arteries

Short Cases (SCs)

SC 1

A 67-year-old male:
- Heavy smoker with type II diabetes
- Unknown coronary artery disease
- Severely compromised global LV function at transthoracic echocardiography with inferior wall motion abnormality
- Cardiac MR required for further characterization

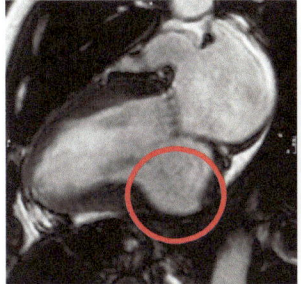 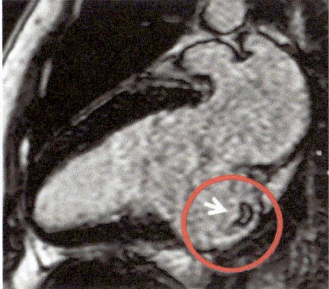

| CINE MR SSFP | T2-weighted STIR | T1-weighted IR TFE post Gad |

There is a focal dilatation of the posterior wall with thinning of the myocardium, transmural late enhancement and a small intracavitary thrombus (→).

 Q1
Differential diagnosis includes:
(Multiple answers might be correct.)
1. Pericardial diverticulum
2. Asymmetric basal dilated cardiomyopathy
3. Posttraumatic inferior wall bulging
4. Inferior wall LV aneurysm
5. Inferior wall LV pseudoaneurysm

3

? Q2

What is the most likely diagnosis?

(Only one option is correct.)

1. Asymmetric basal dilated cardiomyopathy
2. Endocardial diverticulum with thrombus
3. Acute myocardial infarction with microvascular obstruction
4. Chronic post-infarction aneurysm with thrombus
5. Hypertrophic cardiomyopathy

? Q3

What course of action would you take next?

(Multiple answers might be correct.)

1. No need for further imaging or follow-up
2. Surgical excision without follow-up
3. Biopsy
4. Follow-up of the lesion in order to establish indication for further surgery
5. Direct application of an intraventricular patch

CORE

A 38-year-old female:

— With palpitations and shortness of breath on exertion

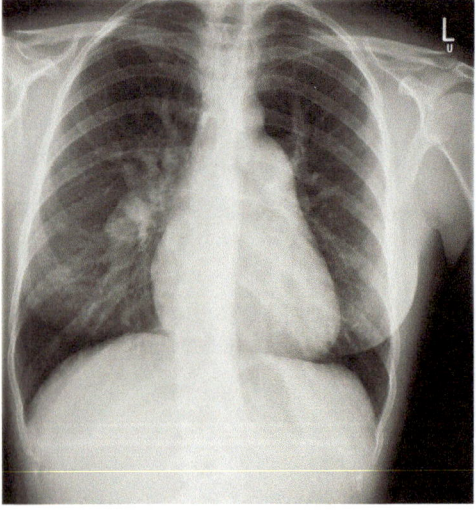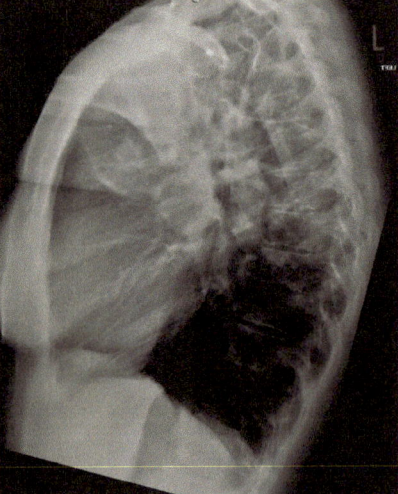

? Q1

Describe the main abnormal findings in the chest plain films.

_____

_____

_____

? Q2

■ Video 3.1

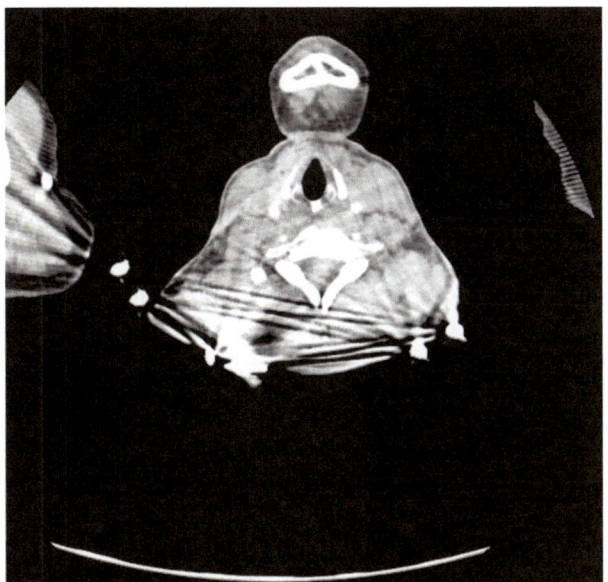

List the four most important abnormal findings in the CT.

_____

_____

_____

? Q3

List four possible causes of increased pulmonary blood flow (in general, not specific to this case).

_____

_____

_____

3

 Q4
Can you identify any cause or causes of increased pulmonary blood flow in this patient?

_____

_____

_____

Answers

Multiple Response Questions (MRQs)

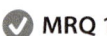 **MRQ 1**
2 and 3
Explanation
Most coronary anomalies are clinically silent. ALCAPA (formerly Bland–White–Garland syndrome) describes a rare coronary anomaly with origin of the left main stem artery from the pulmonary artery.

Primary anomalies of coronary vasculature have an incidence of 1–2% in the general population. There is a varying relation of sudden cardiac death due to coronary anomalies especially those which course between the root of the aorta and the pulmonary artery ranging from 19% to almost 33% in healthy young individuals. A retroaortic course, i.e. between the root of the aorta and the left atrium, is a benign course.

✅ **MRQ 2**
1, 2 and 3
Explanation
The Diamond and Forrester Score has shown to equal other well-established and more complex risk scores in terms of diagnostic accuracy. With this score, patients with a low pretest probability (PTP) should have no further diagnostic workup; patients with an intermediate PTP should be referred for noninvasive stress testing, and patients with a high PTP should be considered for invasive coronary angiography.

✅ **MRQ 3**
2, 3 and 5
Explanation
The images show an acute pulmonary embolism with saddle emboli in the central pulmonary arteries and centrally located filling defect subsegmentally. CT angiography of the pulmonary arteries is regarded as first-line imaging modality in case of suspected acute PE. MR imaging may be performed as an alternative method in patients who cannot undergo contrast-enhanced CT pending sufficient expertise in pulmonary MR angiography.

Short Cases (SCs)

SC 1

✅ **Q1**

4 and 5

✅ **Q2**

4

✅ **Q3**

4

Explanation

The cine and LGE images show a transmural ischemic late enhancement with infe-rior LV aneurysm as a sequelae after myocardial infarction. There is no myocardial oedema; therefore, this is not an acute myocardial infarction, and we see a chronic scar. Due to slow flow, an intracavitary thrombus has developed.

CMR features: Transmural late enhancement with no signs of oedema. There is a continuity of ventricular wall allowing the differentiation of the abnormality from pseudoaneurysms (myocardial rupture contained by pericardial adhesions and thrombus formation).

CORE

✅ **Q1**

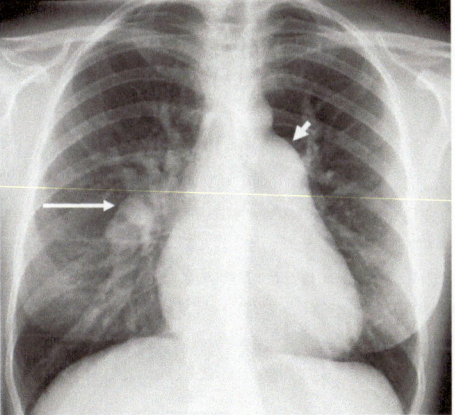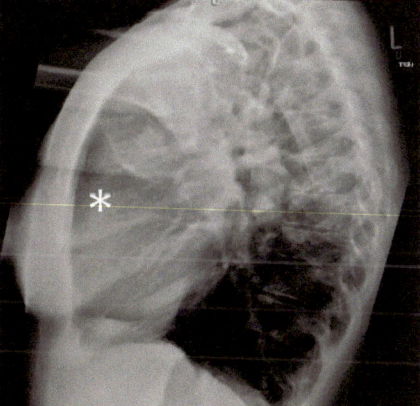

- — Pulmonary hypertension findings (enlarged pulmonary artery, pruning of peripheral arterioles)
- — Right ventricular enlargement

Explanation

Radiographic findings of pulmonary hypertension. Frontal chest radiograph shows a prominent main pulmonary artery (short arrow), dilated right interlobar artery

3

(long arrow) and pruning of peripheral pulmonary vascularity. Lateral chest radiograph shows filling of the retrosternal airspace (asterisk), a result of right ventricular dilatation.

 Q2

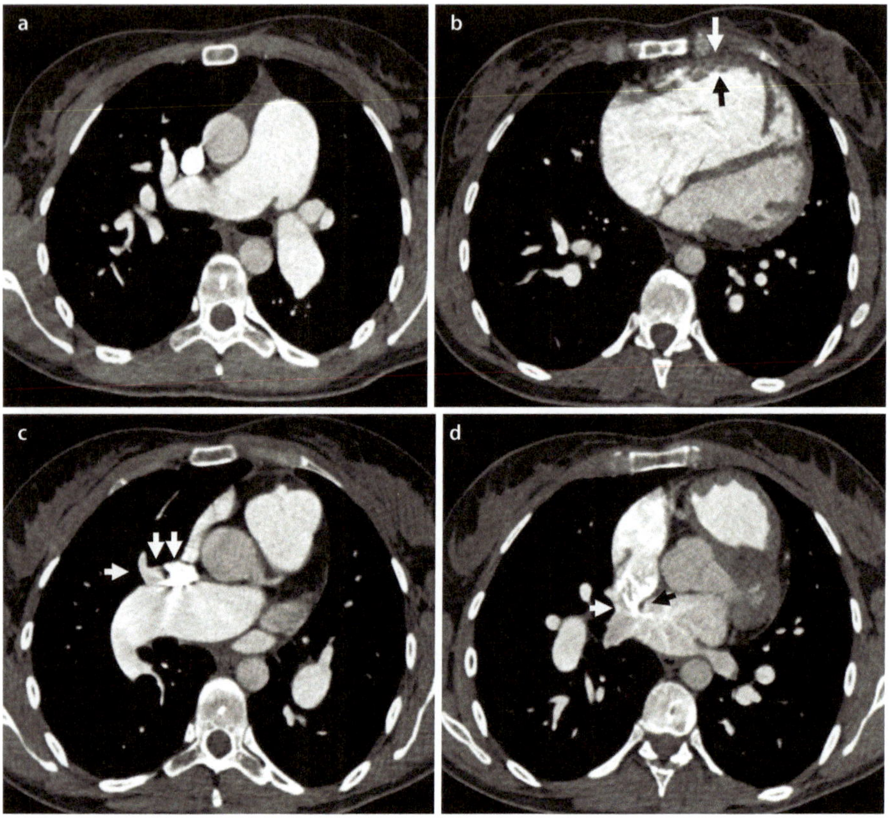

![CT images a, b, c, d]

- **Image (A)** Dilatation of the pulmonary trunk (larger than the adjacent ascending aorta) and main pulmonary artery
- **Image (B)** Dilatation of the right ventricle and hypertrophy of the right ventricular myocardium indicating an increased pressure in the pulmonary arterial system (arrows)
- **Image (C)** Anomalous drainage of the right superior pulmonary vein into the superior vena cava (arrows)
- **Image (D)** Atrial septal defect (sinus venosus defect) (arrow)
- Contrast reflux to the inferior vena cava consistent with tricuspid regurgitation

✅ **Q3**

1. Atrial septal defect
2. Ventricular septal defect
3. Anomalous pulmonary venous return
4. Patent ductus arteriosus
5. Atrioventricular canal defect

✅ **Q4**

Correct answer: Anomalous drainage of the right superior pulmonary vein into the superior vena cava and an associated atrial septal defect (sinus venosus defect).
Explanation

The plain film shows an enlargement of the pulmonary trunk and pulmonary arteries. There are also signs of pulmonary hypertension due to pruning of the peripheral pulmonary arteries. There is enlargement of the right heart; the left heart is not dilated. There is no hyperaemia of the lungs detectable.

The CT confirms the signs of pulmonary hypertension and allows us to determine the cause, an atrial septal defect and anomalous pulmonary venous return. This patient has a pulmonary hypertension due to long-standing and uncorrected left-to-right shunt. Consecutively an Eisenmenger's reaction developed leading to pulmonary hypertension and—in the end—to reversal of the shunt (presumably now right-to-left shunt). These information/findings are in so far important, as a correction of the ASD and the partial anomalous return of the right pulmonary veins would lead to a further deterioration of the patient's clinical condition.

Some congenital systemic-to-pulmonary shunts may be diagnosed at CT pulmonary angiography. Although most intracardiac shunts (e.g. atrial septal and ventricular septal defects) are identified at echocardiography, some left-to-right shunts such as sinus venosus defects, patent ductus arteriosus and anomalous pulmonary venous return may be missed; thus, familiarity with their imaging appearances is important.

Literature

Carter BW, Benveniste MF, Madan R, et al. ITMIG classification of mediastinal compartments and multidisciplinary approach to mediastinal masses. Radiographics. 2017;37(2):413–36.

Carter BW, Lichtenberger JP, Benveniste MK, de Groot PM, Wu CC, Erasmus JJ, Truong MT. Revisions to the TNM staging of lung cancer: rationale, significance, and clinical application. Radiographics. 2018;38(2):374–91.

Chen Y-A, Nguyen ET, Dennie C, Wald RM, Crean AM, Yoo S-J, Jiménez-Juan L. Computed tomography and magnetic resonance imaging of the coronary sinus: anatomic variants and congenital anomalies. Insights Imaging. 2014;5(5):547–57.

Etesami M, Ashwath R, Kanne J, Gilkeson RC, Rajiah P. Computed tomography in the evaluation of vascular rings and slings. Insights Imaging. 2014;5(4):507–21.

O'Brien JP, Srichai MB, Hecht EM, Kim DC, Jacobs JE. Anatomy of the heart at multidetector CT: what the radiologist needs to know. Radiographics. 2017;27(6):1569–82.

Oikonomou A, Prassopoulos P. Mimics in chest disease: interstitial opacities. Insights Imaging. 2013;4(1):9–27.

Snoeckx A, Reyntiens P, Desbuquoit D, Spinhoven MJ, Van Schil PE, van Meerbeeck JP, Parizel PM. Evaluation of the solitary pulmonary nodule: size matters, but do not ignore the power of morphology. Insights Imaging. 2018;9(1):73–86.

3

Additional EDiR Preparatory Materials

http://learn.myesr.org

Chest/Thorax Radiology

Electronic supplementary material   The online version of this chapter
(https://doi.org/10.1007/978-3-030-20066-4_4) contains supplementary material,
which is available to authorized users.

4

Multiple Response Questions (MRQs)

? **MRQ 1**
Regarding the anatomy of the airways, which of the following statements are correct?
(Multiple answers might be correct.)
1. The left main bronchus is wider and more vertical than the right main bronchus
2. The posterior aspect of the trachea is formed of cartilage
3. The trachea usually bifurcates at the level of T4/5
4. The left main bronchus lies below the left pulmonary artery
5. The lingular segmental bronchus forms part of the left lower lobe

? **MRQ 2**
Regarding large airway instability (malacia) in chronic obstructive pulmonary disease (COPD), which of the following statements are correct?
(Multiple answers might be correct.)
1. Tracheobronchomalacia usually affects the whole trachea in the same manner
2. Lobar and segmental airways can be affected by instability
3. Excessive dynamic airway collapse is characterised by a bowing of the posterior membrane of the trachea
4. Airway instability is typically diagnosed and graded by spirometry
5. Airway instability is considered to be underdiagnosed in advanced COPD

? **MRQ 3**
Among patients who have solitary pulmonary nodule on their screening CT scan, please specify what are the factors which are associated with a higher risk for cancer:
(Multiple answers might be correct.)
1. Spiculation
2. Older age
3. Existence of interstitial lung disease
4. Male gender
5. Upper lobes

? **MRQ 4**
Regarding chest radiograph, pneumothorax is located in supine position mainly:
(Only one option is correct.)
1. Ventral
2. Basal
3. Lateral
4. Dorsal
5. Apical

MRQ 5

Regarding interstitial lung disease, which of the following statements are correct?
(Multiple answers might be correct.)

1. Cryptogenic organising pneumonia (COP) may present with CT findings similar to that of chronic eosinophilic pneumonia
2. Ground glass opacities are commonly seen in non-specific interstitial pneumonitis (NSIP)
3. Cryptogenic organising pneumonia (COP) is associated with cigarette smoking
4. In patients with subacute hypersensitivity pneumonitis (HP), centrilobular nodules can be seen
5. In the fibrotic phase of acute respiratory distress syndrome (ARDS), changes are most severe in the dependent part of the lungs

MRQ 6

A 57-year-old male.

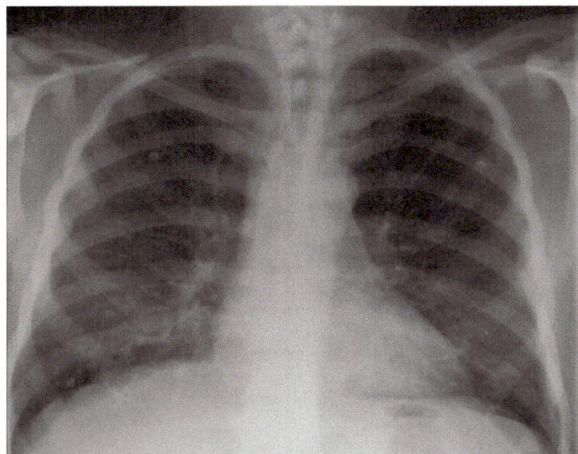

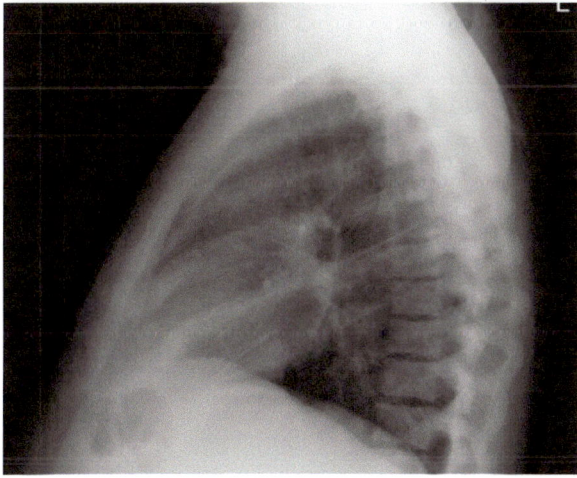

What is the most likely diagnosis?
(Only one option is correct.)
1. Metastatic prostate carcinoma
2. Normal/normal variant
3. Sickle cell disease
4. Paget's disease
5. Metastatic rectal carcinoma

4   ❓ MRQ 7
Asymptomatic patient.

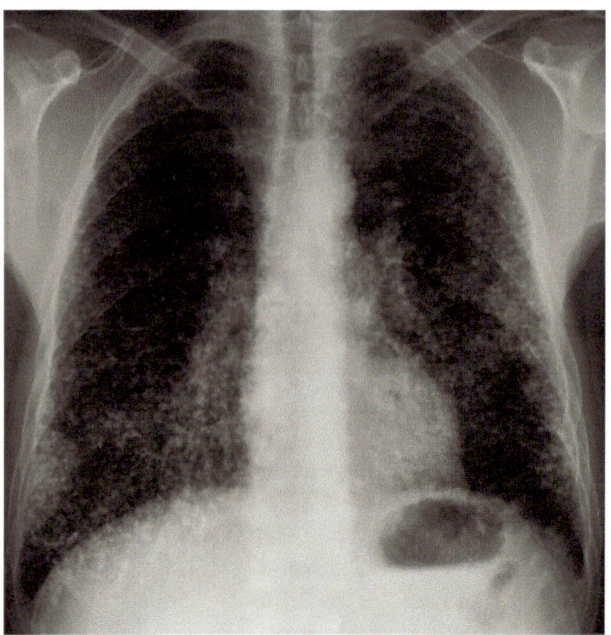

What is the most likely diagnosis?
(Only one option is correct.)
1. Alveolar septal amyloidosis
2. Sarcoidosis
3. Acute miliary tuberculosis
4. Alveolar microlithiasis
5. Silicosis

? MRQ 8
Blunt thoracic trauma.

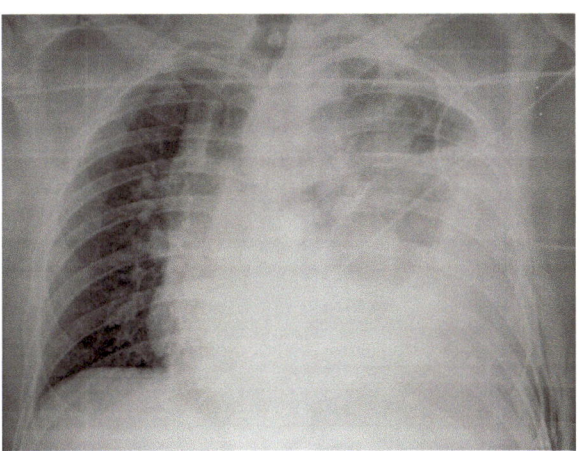

Regarding this bedside chest X-ray, which are the correct answers?
(Multiple answers might be correct.)
1. Right displacement of the mediastinum
2. Possible left pleural effusion
3. Large right pleural effusion
4. Left upper lobe pulmonary consolidation
5. Left subcutaneous emphysema

Short Cases (SCs)

SC 1

A 29-year-old patient:
- With incidental haemoptysis and right lower lobe opacity on the chest radiograph
- Contrast-enhanced CT in the arterial phase (mediastinal and lung window) is performed

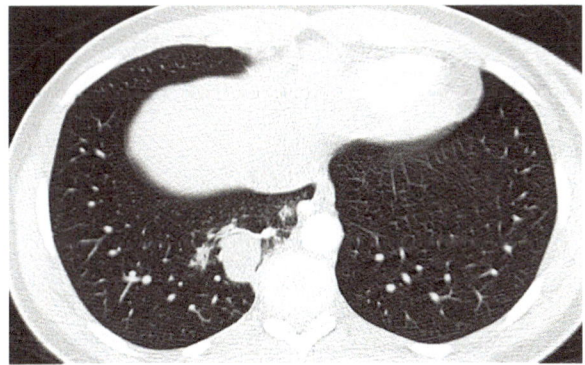

4

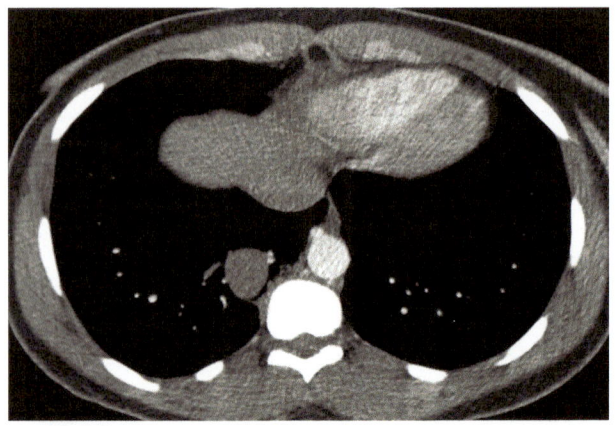

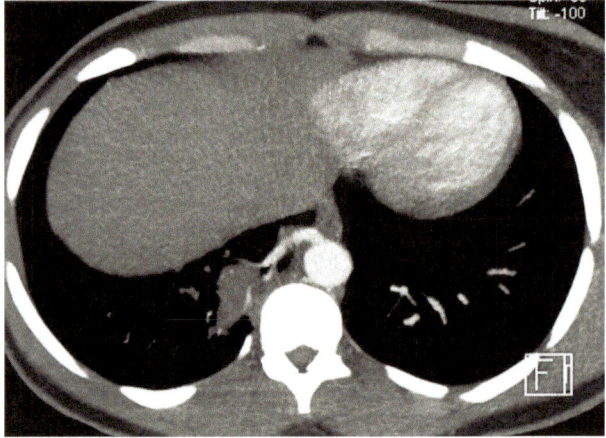

? **Q1**
Indicate the abnormality.

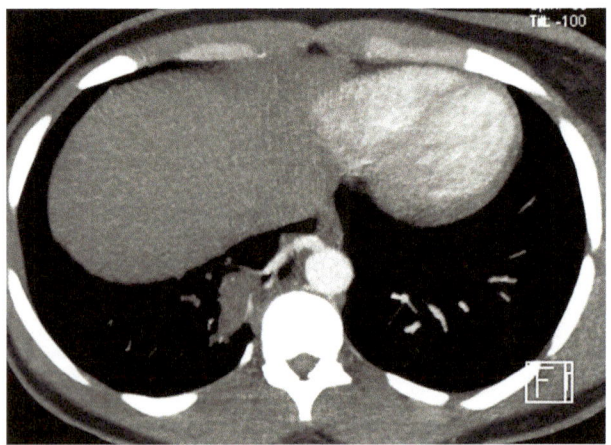

? Q2

Differential diagnosis includes:

(Multiple answers might be correct.)

1. Pneumonia
2. Carcinoid tumour
3. Congenital cystic adenomatoid malformation
4. Pulmonary sequestration
5. Arteriovenous malformation

? Q3

Give the most likely diagnosis.

_____

_____

_____

? Q4

What is the best course of action?

(Only one option is correct.)

1. PET/CT
2. Embolisation
3. CT-guided biopsy
4. Surgery
5. Transesophageal ultrasound

SC 2

A 72-year-old female:
- With known chronic obstructive pulmonary disease (COPD)
- CT is requested due to decreasing lung function

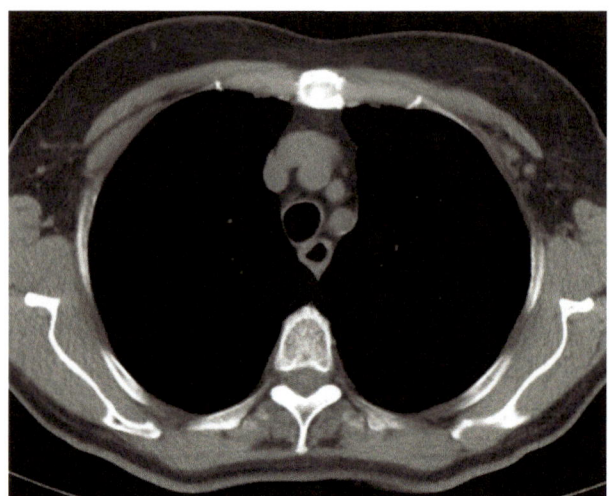

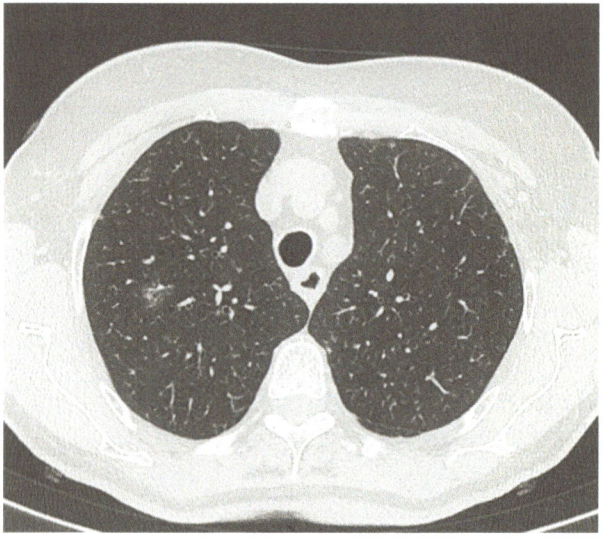

? Q1
Indicate the abnormality.

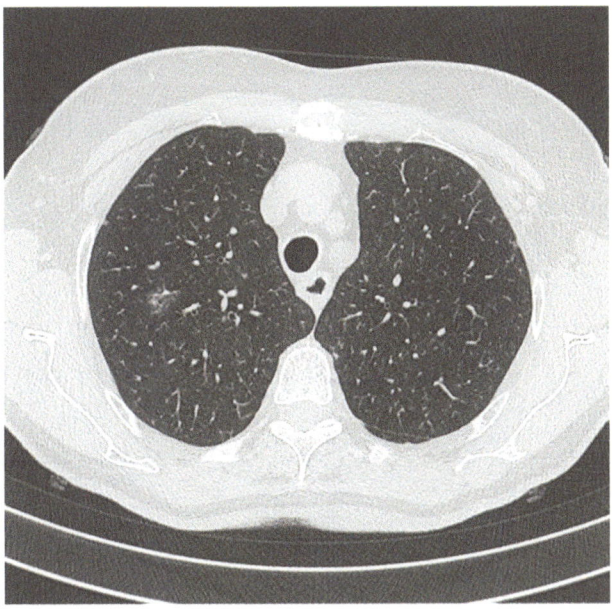

? Q2
The findings are lesions that:
(Multiple answers might be correct.)
1. It is a sub-solid nodule
2. It does not need imaging follow-up
3. It needs immediate surgery
4. It needs imaging follow-up
5. It needs to be admitted for lung biopsy

? Q3

4

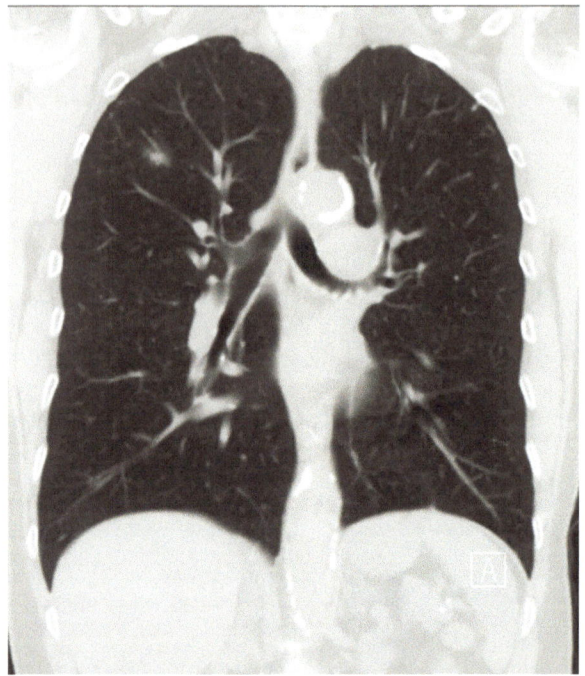

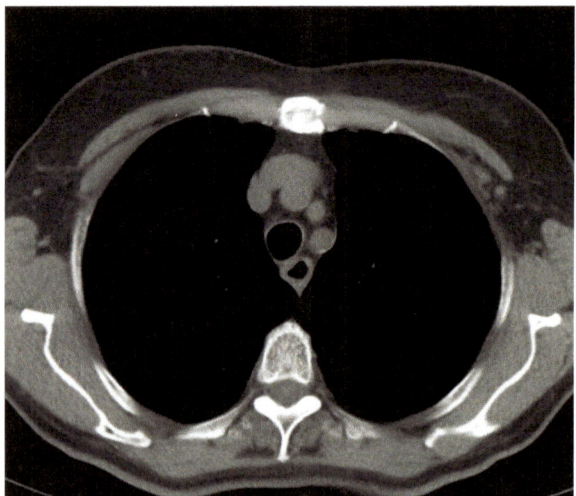

Based on images alone, these findings could be:
(Multiple answers might be correct.)
1. Pneumonia
2. Hamartoma
3. Aspergilloma
4. Adenocarcinoma in situ
5. Area of localised pulmonary haemorrhage

Q4
CT performed 3 years later:

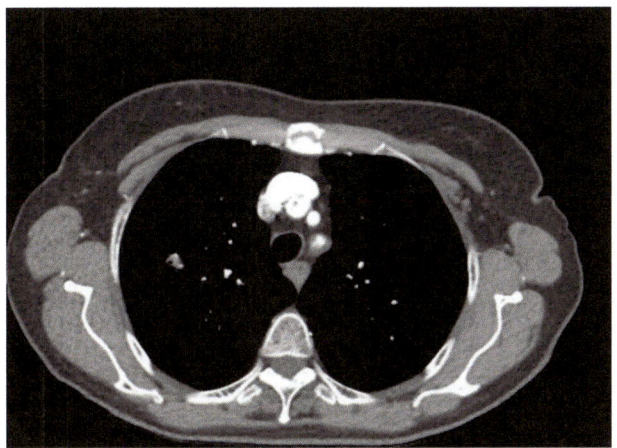

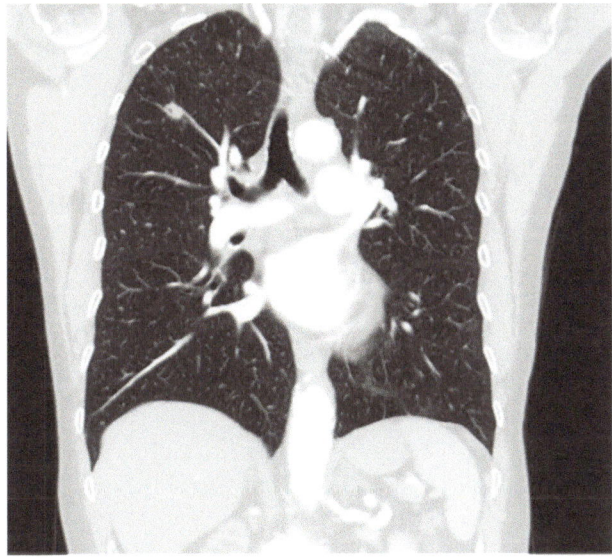

What does this CT show?
(Multiple answers might be correct.)

1. A part-solid lesion
2. Growth
3. Enlarged lymph nodes
4. Cavitation
5. No change

Q5
Give the most likely diagnosis.

_____

_____

_____

4

SC 3

A 67-year-old male:
- Previous cardiac surgery
- Admitted with infection of unknown origin
- Routine chest radiograph is performed

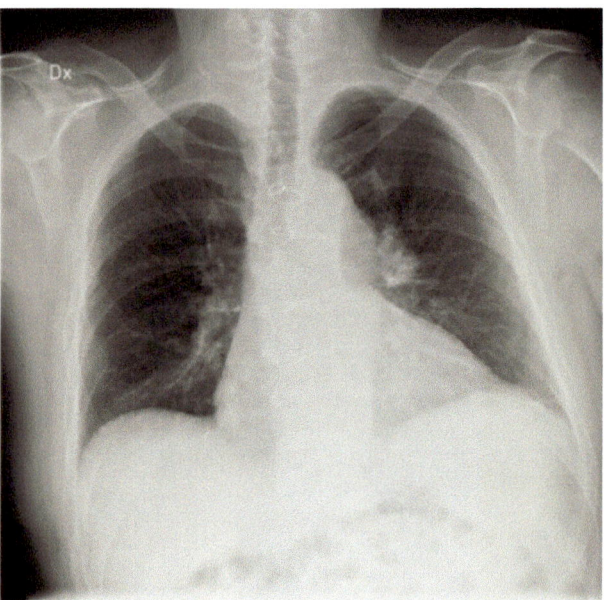

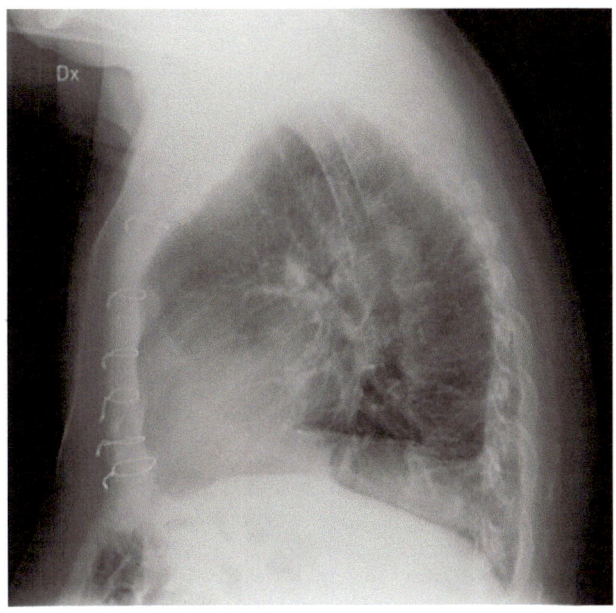

❓ Q1
Indicate the abnormality.

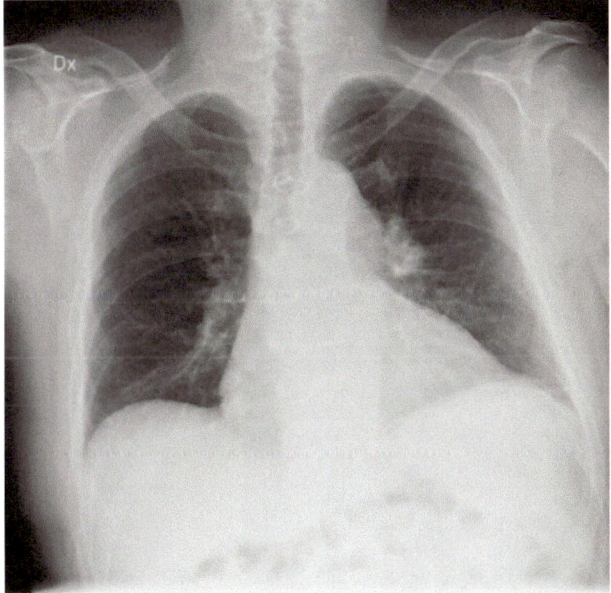

? Q2

What course of action would you take next?

(Multiple answers might be correct.)

1. Suggest a bronchoscopy
2. Suggest a control chest radiograph in 6 weeks
3. Suggest a CT of the thorax and abdomen
4. Suggest a CT of the thorax
5. Suggest testing for tuberculosis

4

? Q3

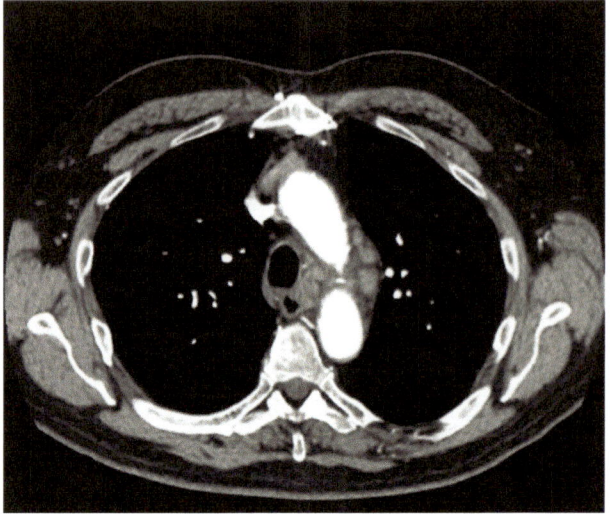

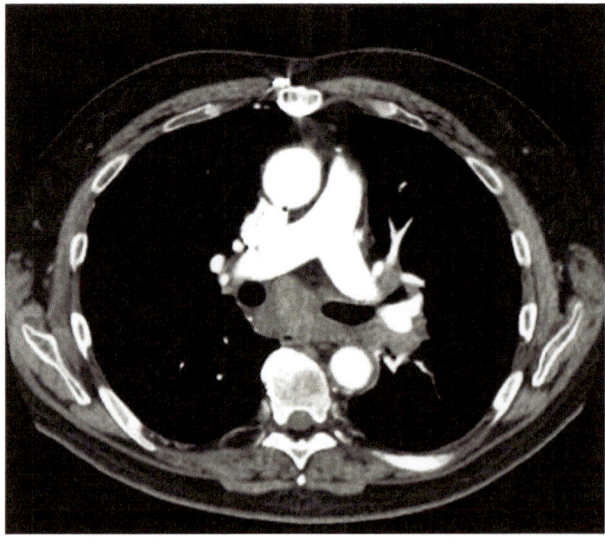

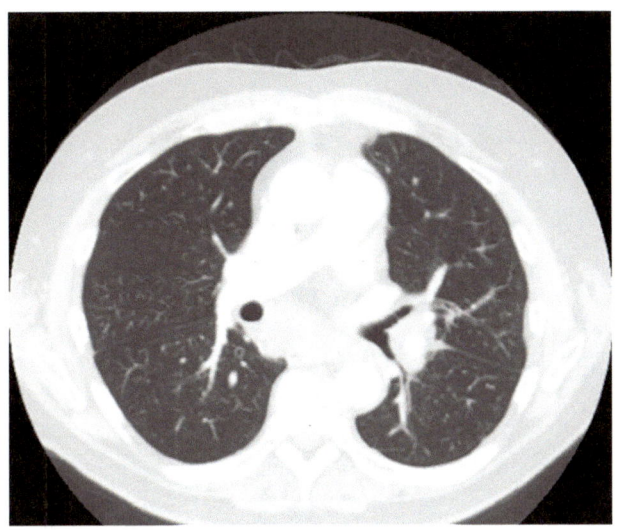

Differential diagnosis includes:
(Multiple answers might be correct.)
1. Lymphoma
2. Paraganglioma
3. Carcinoid tumour
4. Mediastinal abscess
5. Broncogenic cyst

CORE

A 60-year-old lady:
- With cough and loss of weight the last 6 months

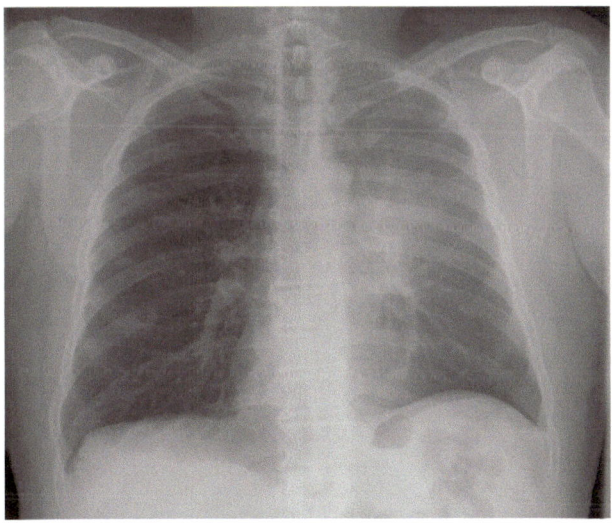

4

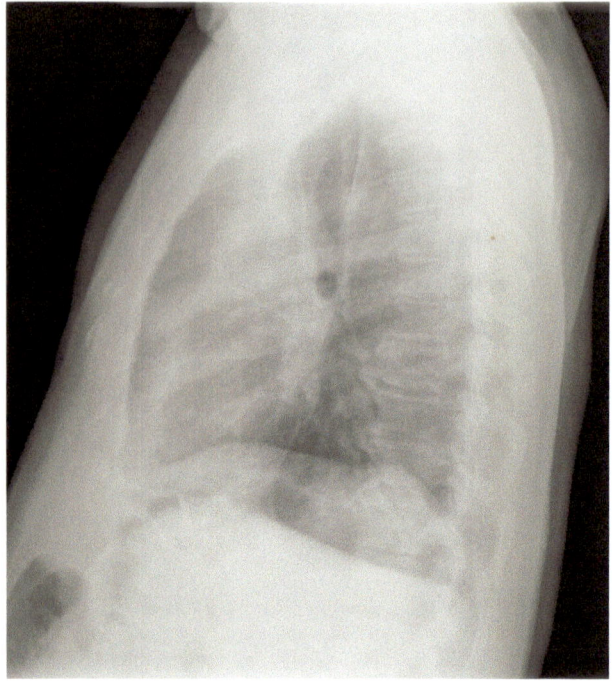

❓ Q1

Describe the major findings on the PA and lateral images, and list the radiological signs that lead to this conclusion.

_____

_____

_____

Q2

- **Video 4.1**

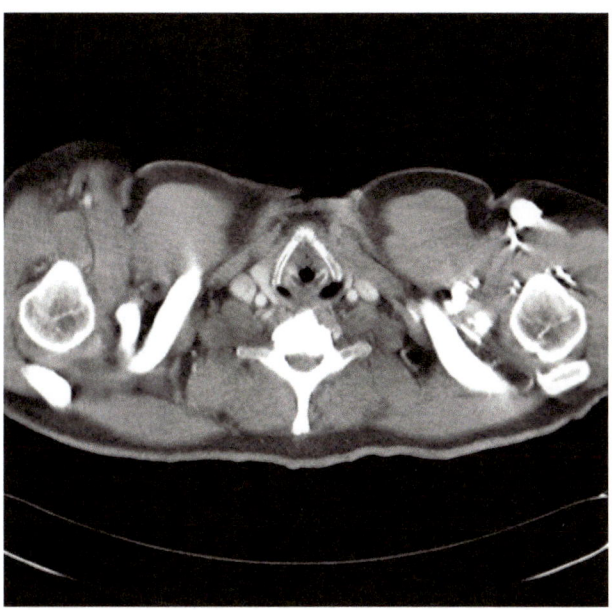

- **Video 4.2**

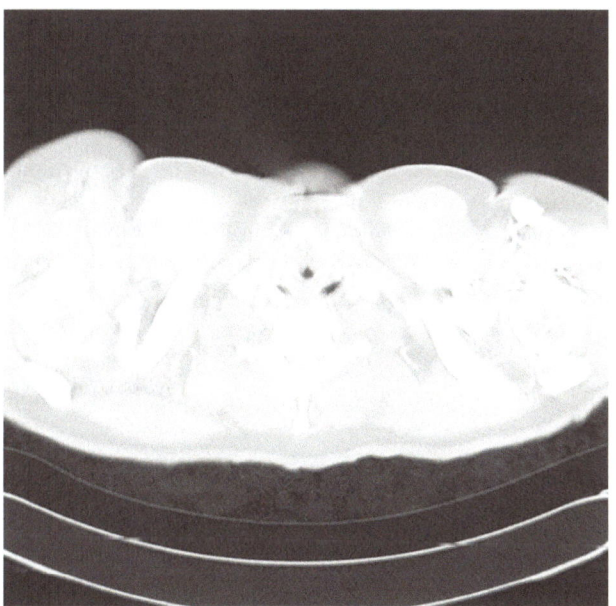

List the significant abnormalities.

_____

_____

_____

? Q3
What is the most likely diagnosis?

_____

_____

_____

Answers

Multiple Response Questions (MRQs)

✓ **MRQ 1**
3 and 4

✓ **MRQ 2**
2, 3 and 5

✓ **MRQ 3**
1, 2, 3 and 5
Explanation
Marginal spiculation has been known for many years to be associated with malignancy.
The relationship between age and lung cancer risk has been clearly established, with an accelerating increase in risk associated with advancing age. The existence of an interstitial lung disease particularly idiopathic pulmonary fibrosis is also associated with an increased risk of cancer. Lung cancers occur more frequently in the upper lobes, with a predilection for the right lung.

✓ **MRQ 4**
1

✓ **MRQ 5**
1, 2 and 4

✓ **MRQ 6**
1

MRQ 7

4

Explanation

Alveolar microlithiasis (AM) is an idiopathic accumulation of tiny calculi (microliths) within alveolar spaces. The chest plain film is characteristic of AM, showing multiple micronodules, most severe in the middle and lower lung zones, with characteristic calcium density; the absence of symptoms is also an important clue.

MRQ 8

1, 2, 4 and 5

Short Cases (SCs)

SC 1

Q1

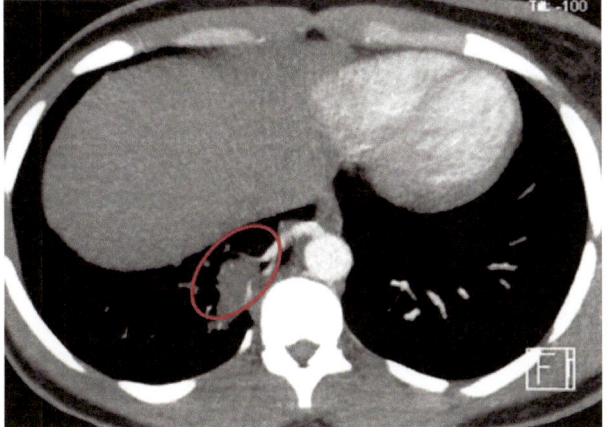

Q2

4

Q3

Pulmonary sequestration

Q4

4

Explanation

Pulmonary sequestration is a portion of lung detached from the remaining normal lung, typically presenting as homogeneous opacity or as a cystic mass. Most frequently occurs in the lower lobes. A confident diagnosis can be made by demonstrating the systemic arterial supply on contrast-enhanced CT or with MRI.

SC 2

✅ **Q1**

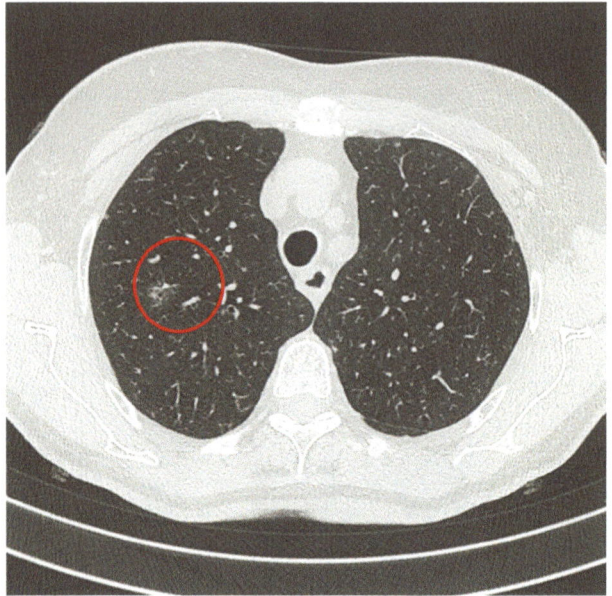

✅ **Q2**
1 and 4

✅ **Q3**
1, 4 and 5

✅ **Q4**
1 and 2

✅ **Q5**
Adenocarcinoma

SC 3

 Q1

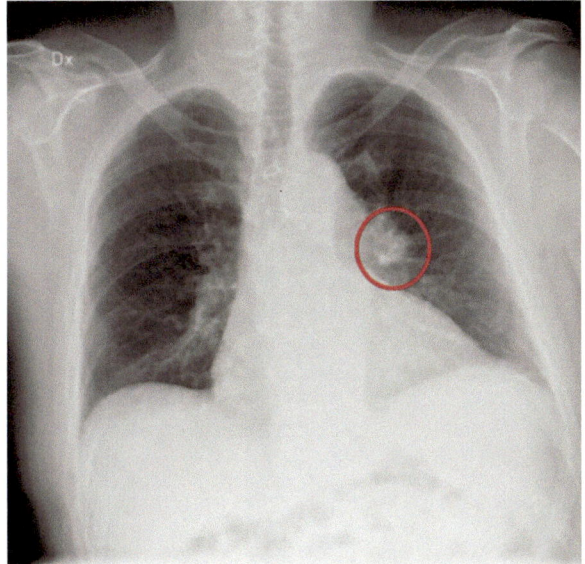

 Q2
3

 Q3
1

CORE

 Q1

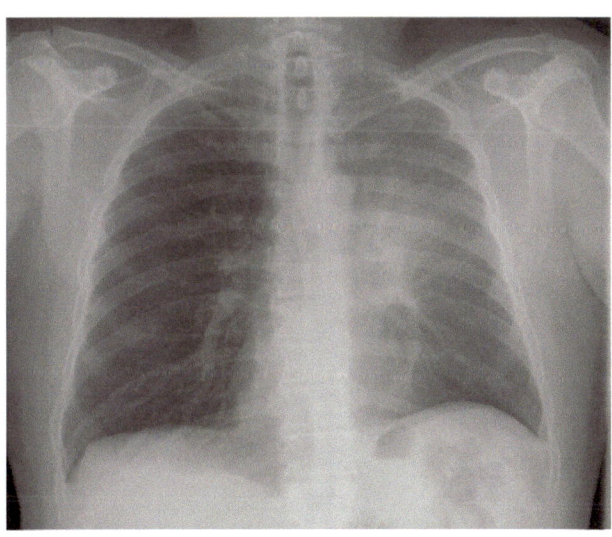

4

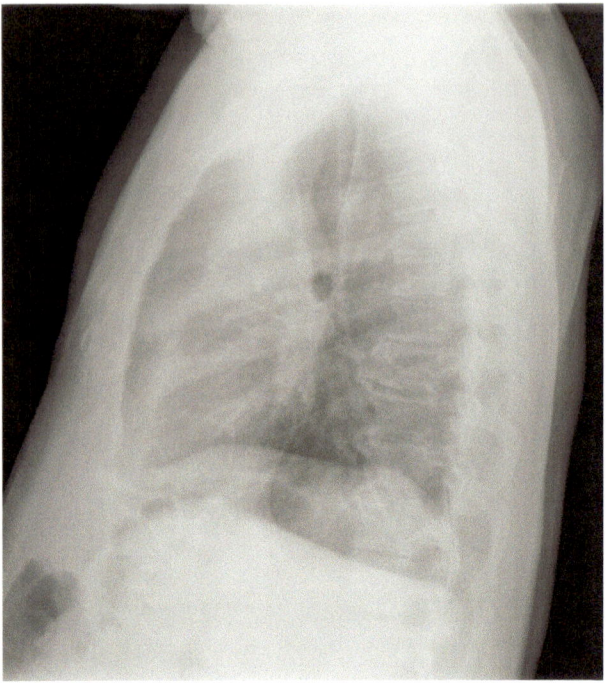

Posteroanterior chest film showing an increased opacity in the left hemithorax extending from the hilum and fading laterally and inferiorly. This opacity causes obliteration of the left upper mediastinal and cardiac border. The lateral edge of this opacity is ill-defined. Lateral chest film demonstrates a retrosternal opacity with a sharply defined posterior border due to anteriorly displaced major fissure (arrows). These signs suggest a left upper lobe collapse.

Left upper lobe collapses anteriorly and medially, and the major fissure (arrow-heads in the scheme) is displaced medially and forward in a plane roughly parallel to the anterior chest wall.

✅ Q2

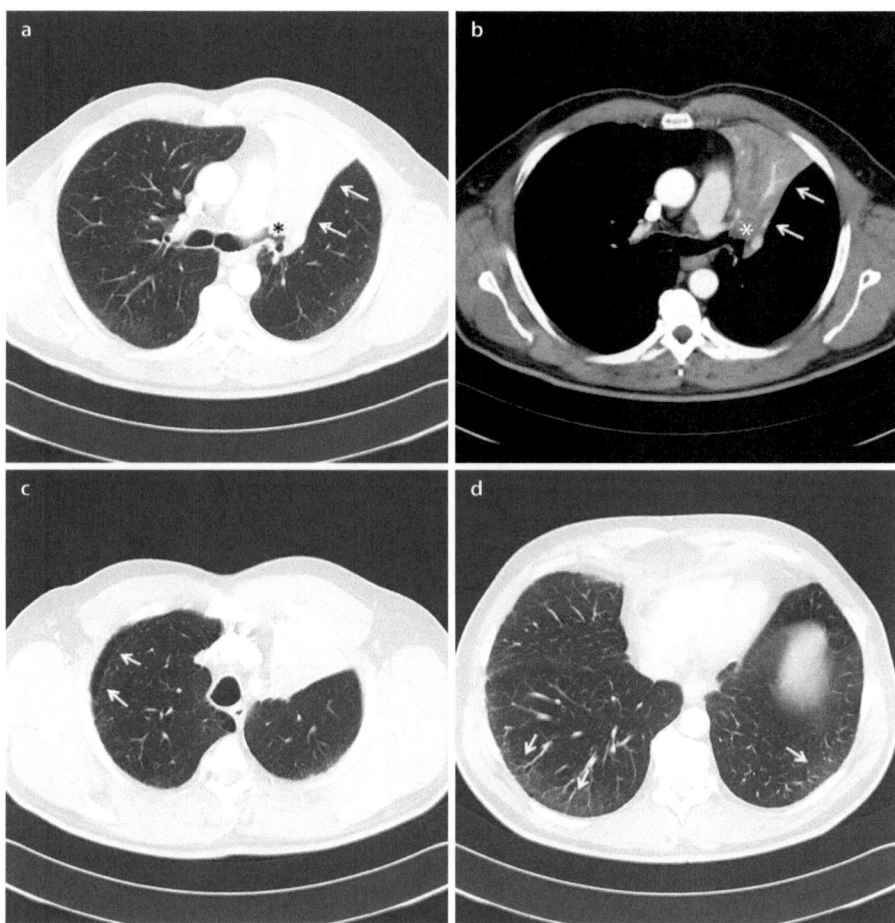

Chest CT scans confirm the left upper lobe collapse. Note the forward displacement of the left oblique fissure (arrows in A, B) and mediastinal shift to the left. Presence of a left hilar mass with resulting occlusion of the left upper and lingular bronchus (asterisk in A, B). Axial CT images showing paraseptal and centrilobular emphysema (arrows in C) in upper lobes and minimal subpleural reticulation and ground glass opacities in the lower lobes suggesting fibrotic changes (arrows in D).

✅ Q3
Bronchogenic carcinoma.

Literature

Ceylan N, Bayraktaroglu S, Savaş R, Alper H. CT findings of high attenuation pulmonary abnormalities. Insights into Imaging. 2010;1(4):287–92.

Lee EY, Boiselle PM, Cleveland RH. Multidetector CT evaluation of congenital lung anomalies. Radiology. 2008;247(3):632–48.

MacMahon H, Naidich DP, Goo JM, et al. Guidelines for Management of Incidental Pulmonary Nodules Detected on CT images: from the Fleischner Society. Radiology. 2017 July;284(1):228–43.

Marini TJ, He K, Hobbs SK, Kaproth-Joslin K. Pictorial review of the pulmonary vasculature: from arteries to veins. Insights into Imaging. 2018;9(6):971–87.

Nin CS, de Souza VV, do Amaral RH, et al. Thoracic lymphadenopathy in benign diseases: a state of the art review. Respir Med. 2016;112:10–7.

Nishino M, Itoh H, Hatabu H. A practical approach to high-resolution CT of diffuse lung disease. Eur J Radiol. 2014;83(1):6–19.

Rossi SE, Erasmus JJ, McAdams HP, Sporn TA, Goodman PC. Pulmonary drug toxicity: radiologic and pathologic manifestations. Radiographics. 2000;20(5):1245–59.

Shepard JO, Flores EJ, Abbott GB. Imaging of the trachea. Ann Cardiothorac Surg. 2018;7(2):197–209.

Additional EDiR Preparatory Materials

http://learn.myesr.org

EDiR Preparatory Sessions

http://learn.myesr.org
Pulmonary vascular disease.
Chest trauma.
Lung infection in the immunocompromised host.

Genitourinary Radiology

Electronic supplementary material   The online version of this chapter
(https://doi.org/10.1007/978-3-030-20066-4_5) contains supplementary material,
which is available to authorized users.

Multiple Response Questions (MRQs)

? MRQ 1

A 43-year-old woman presents with abdominal pain:

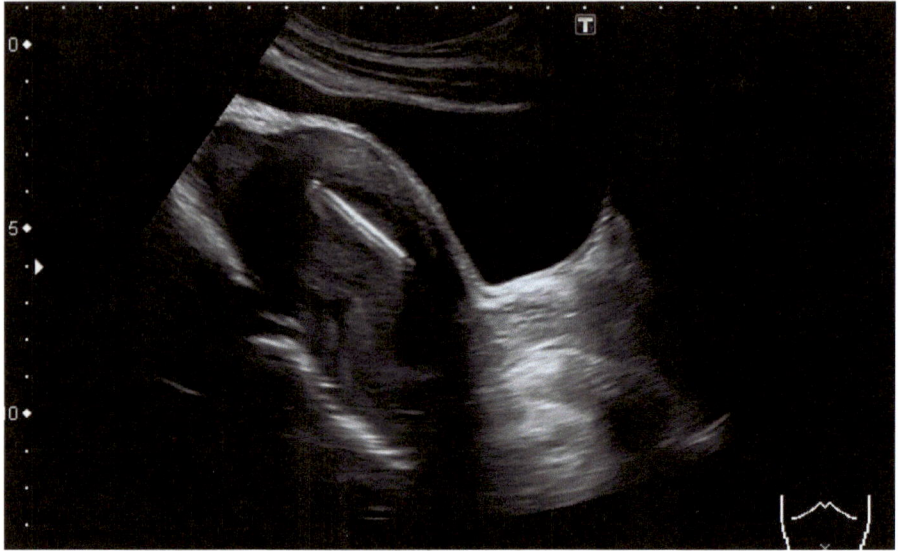

Which of the following statements are correct?

(Multiple answers might be correct.)

1. The appearances are typical of an endometrial polyp
2. The appearances are associated with an increased risk of pelvic inflammatory disease
3. The appearances are typical of adenomyosis
4. The appearances are typical of an intrauterine contraceptive device
5. The appearances are associated with an increased risk of ectopic pregnancy

MRQ 2
Unenhanced CT in a 58-year-old woman with malaise and a palpable abdominal mass:

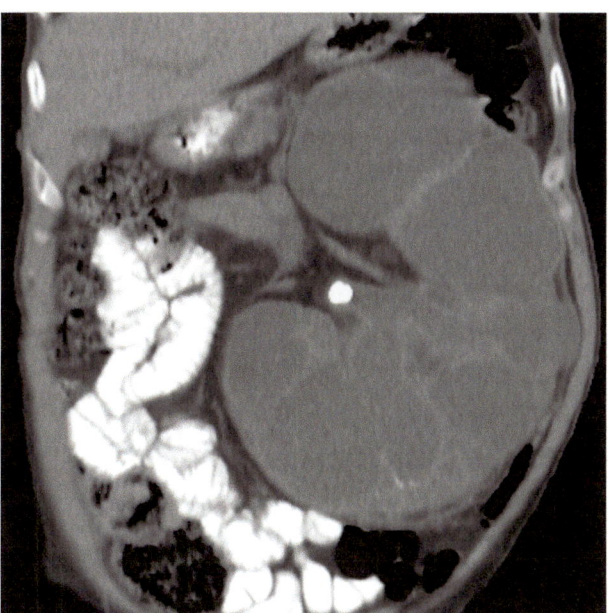

What is the most likely diagnosis?
(Only one option is correct.)
1. Polycystic kidney disease
2. Xanthogranulomatous pyelonephritis
3. Renal tuberculosis
4. Renal aspergillosis
5. Pyonephrosis

MRQ 3
Which of the following statements about renal cancer are correct?
(Multiple answers might be correct.)
1. Most common differentials for lesions showing density 40–70 HU at unenhanced CT are renal cancer, oncocytoma and adenoma
2. Papillary and chromophobe renal cancers are more frequent than clear cell carcinoma
3. CT or MRI cannot differentiate with certainty oncocytomas and lipid-poor angiomyolipomas from renal cancer
4. On unenhanced CT, homogeneous lesions of density > 70 HU are most often due to haemorrhagic cysts
5. The majority of angiomyolipomas are lipid poor

? MRQ 4

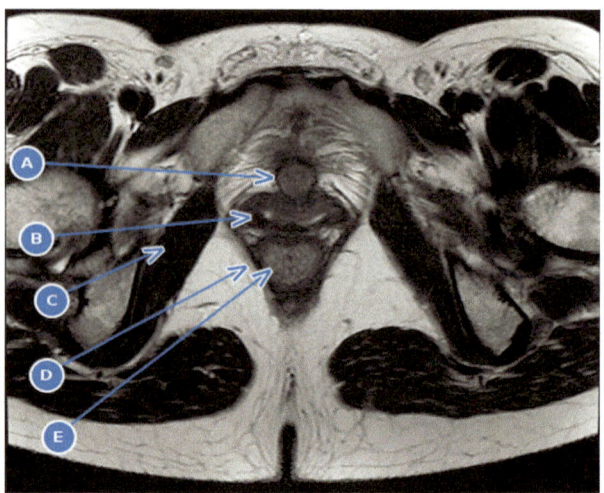

Annotate the labelled areas in this axial MR image of the pelvis:
1. Anus
2. Levator ani muscle
3. Obturator internus muscle
4. Urethra
5. Vagina

? MRQ 5

Regarding uterine leiomyomas on MR imaging, which of the following statements are correct?
(Multiple answers might be correct.)
1. Uterine myomas most typically display low signal intensity on T2WI with hyperintense rim
2. Myomas are typically elliptic in shape with blurry borders
3. Red degeneration of uterine myoma is the most common form of degeneration during pregnancy
4. Uterine myomas most typically display low signal intensity on T1WI with hyperintense rim
5. Pedunculated myoma may require differentiation from ovarian tumour

? MRQ 6

Bosniak classification system of renal cystic masses grade 2F includes:
(Multiple answers might be correct.)
1. Clearly malignant cystic mass or a necrotic component with enhancing soft tissue components
2. Indeterminate cystic masses with thickened irregular septa with enhancement

3. Benign cyst with a few thin septa, which may contain fine calcifications or a small segment of mildly thickened calcification. Lesions less than 3 cm with sharp margins but without enhancement
4. Benign simple cyst with thin wall without septa, calcifications or solid components
5. Renal cysts with multiple thin septa, a septum thicker than hairline, slightly thick wall or with calcification, which may be thick

❓ MRQ 7

In a pregnant patient involved in a road traffic accident with multiple injuries, what would you expect to do?
(Multiple answers might be correct.)
1. In non-life-threatening situations and depending on availability, MRI may be an alternative to protect the foetus from radiation
2. No radiation examinations are performed to protect the foetus
3. All X-ray and CT scans are performed but without contrast enhancement to protect foetus health
4. If in doubt, mother's life first
5. In potential life-threatening injuries, all mandatory X-ray and CT examinations are performed

❓ MRQ 8

Regarding CT imaging of urolithiasis, which of the following statements are true?
(Multiple answers might be correct.)
1. CT is unable to provide the size of urolithic stones
2. A low-dose CT protocol is recommended
3. Although unlikely, fornix rupture may be caused by intravenous contrast media application
4. Stranding around the ureter (swelling of the fat) may be useful in difficult cases
5. If urolithiasis is apparent, CT is able to locate the problem region/height

Short Cases (SCs)

SC 1

A 35-year-old woman:
- She has been with systolic/diastolic hypertension for 10 months
- She is referred to US Doppler evaluation of renal vessels
- It has been impossible to identify the two renal arteries at colour Doppler, and only the kidneys could be examined
- This is the Doppler spectrum at the hilum of the right kidney. Flow signals at the left kidney were normal

5

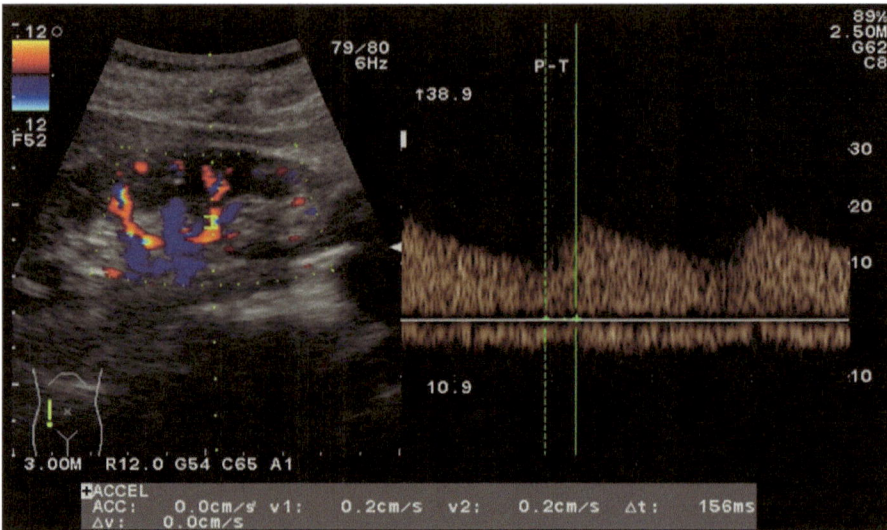

❓ Q1

How would you best describe this Doppler waveform?

(Only one option is correct.)

1. Normal
2. Tardus parvus
3. Accelerated
4. High resistance
5. Turbulent flow

❓ Q2

What haemodynamic condition does this Doppler waveform indicate?

(Only one option is correct.)

1. Normal flow
2. Post stenotic flow
3. Decreased intrarenal resistance
4. Increased intrarenal resistance
5. Increased velocity at renal hilum

? Q3
The patient underwent catheter angiography:

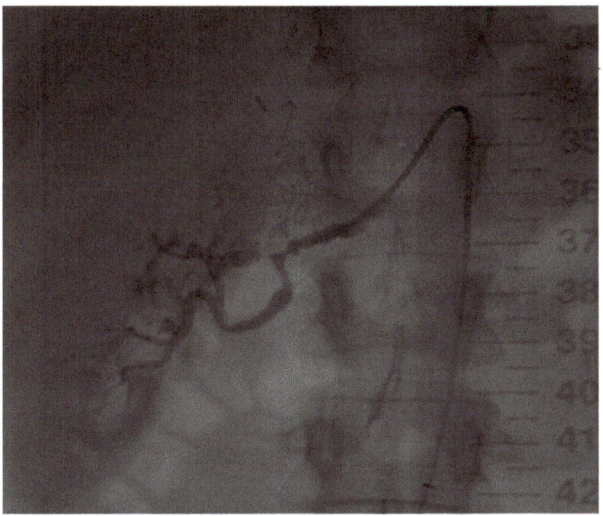

What is the most likely diagnosis?
(Only one option is correct.)
1. Renal artery aneurysm
2. Partial renal infarction
3. Findings suggest vasculitic changes
4. Renal artery stenosis due to atherosclerosis
5. Renal artery stenosis due to fibromuscular dysplasia

? Q4
What would you suggest as first therapeutic approach in this case?
(Only one option is correct.)
1. Antihypertensive medical therapy
2. Open vascular surgery
3. Balloon angioplasty
4. Arterial stenting
5. Renal denervation

5

SC 2

A 67-year-old female:
— Sagittal US image of the abdomen is performed for a palpable mass:

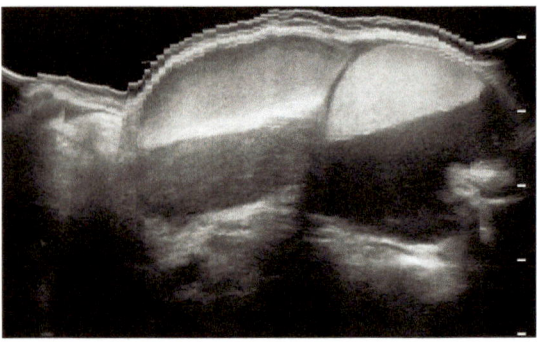

? Q1
Indicate abnormality.

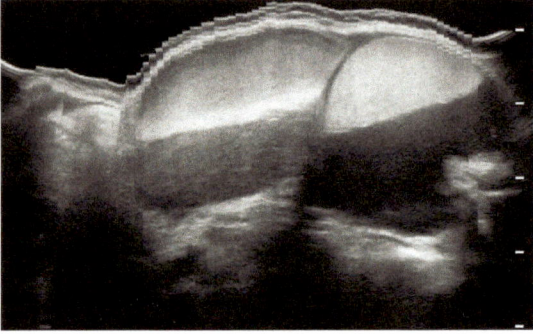

? Q2
Which is the most likely diagnosis?
(Only one option is correct.)
1. A dilated urinary bladder
2. A complicated mesenteric cyst
3. Ascites
4. Ovarian dermoid cyst
5. Non-specific ovarian tumour

? Q3
What could you do to confirm the nature of the lesion?
(Multiple answers might be correct.)
1. Follow-up US
2. MRI
3. US-guided percutaneous biopsy
4. CT
5. Contrast-enhanced US

? Q4
Which is the final diagnosis?
(Only one option is correct.)

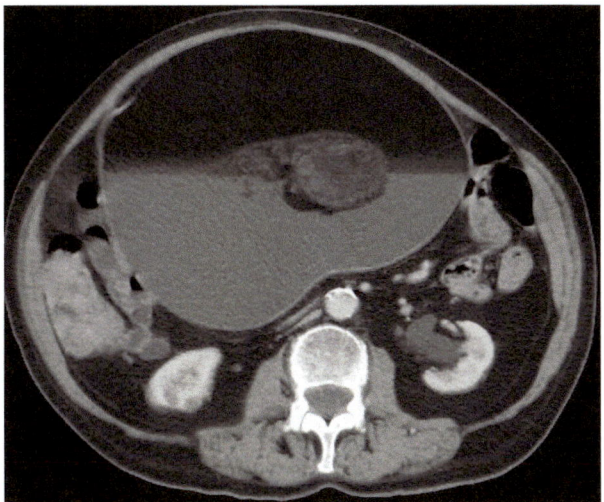

1. Ascites
2. Ovarian dermoid cyst
3. A complicated mesenteric cyst
4. A dilated urinary bladder
5. Non-specific ovarian tumour

? Q5
Which of the following statements about ovarian mature cystic teratomas (dermoid cysts) are correct?
(Multiple answers might be correct.)
1. They affect an older age group than epithelial neoplasms of the ovary
2. They are germ cell tumours of the ovary
3. Most are asymptomatic
4. They are bilateral in 10% of cases
5. They are composed of well-differentiated derivations from one of the three germ layers: endoderm, mesoderm and ectoderm

SC 3

A 46-year-old female patient:
- Heavy menstrual bleeding
- Menstrual periods lasting more than a week
- Pelvic pressure
- Pelvic pain
- Frequent urination
- Backache

5

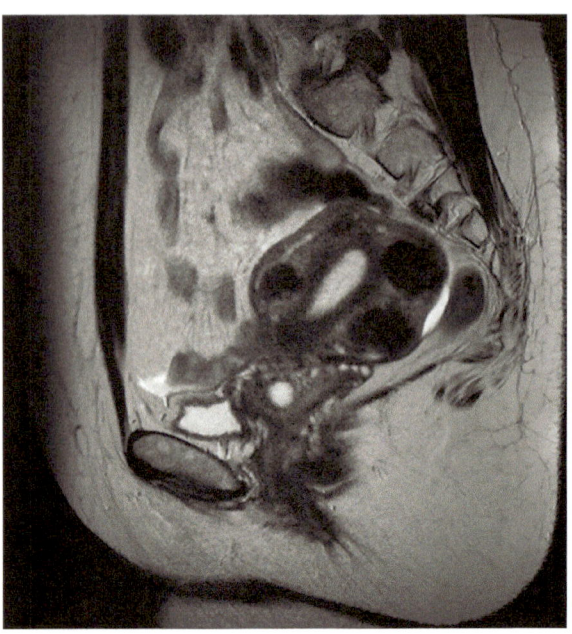

? **Q1**
Indicate the four abnormalities in the uterine body.

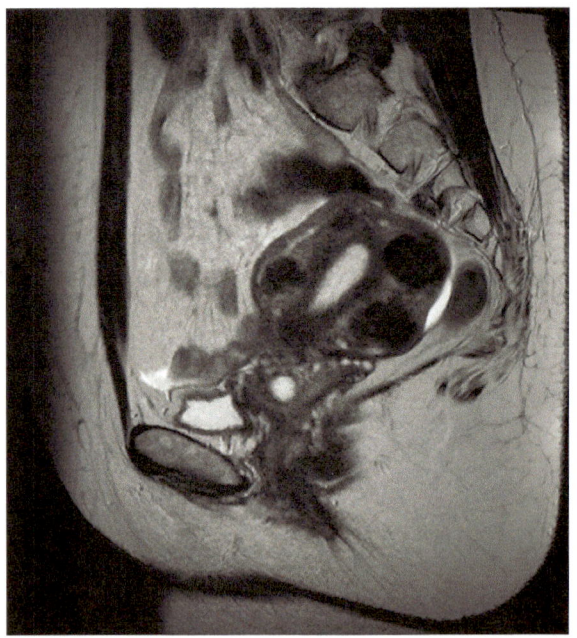

❓ Q2

Indicate the abnormality in the uterine body.

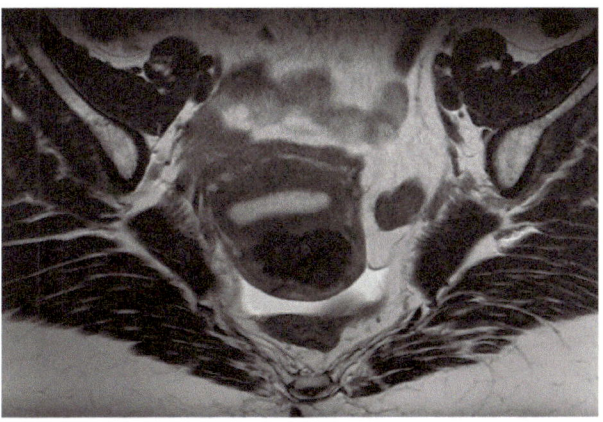

❓ Q3

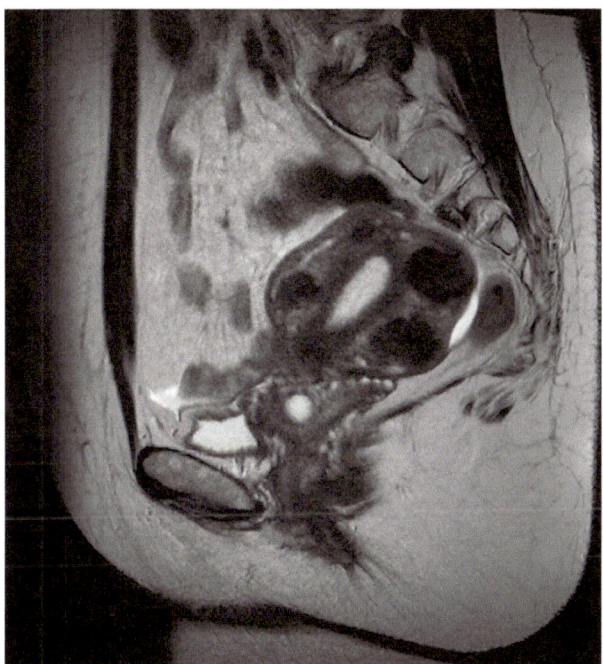

5

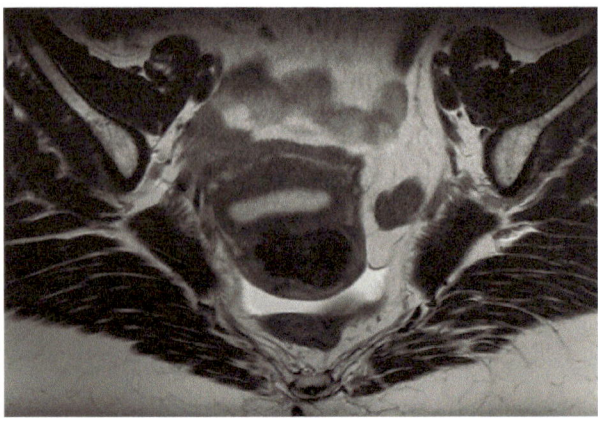

Which radiological findings do you recognise in these MR images?
(Multiple answers might be correct.)
1. Multiple focal lesions within myometrium
2. Retroverted uterus
3. Nabothian cysts
4. Urinary bladder infiltration
5. Trace of fluid in the rectouterine pouch (Douglas' pouch)

 Q4

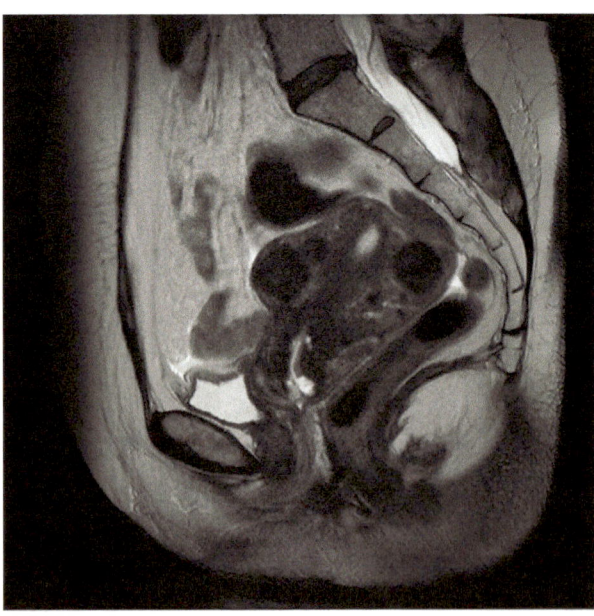

Differential diagnosis includes:
(Multiple answers might be correct.)
1. Urethral diverticulum
2. Endometrial carcinoma
3. Leiomyomas
4. Cervical cancer
5. Nabothian cysts

? Q5
Regarding the lesions of the uterine corpus, give the most likely diagnosis.

_____

_____

_____

CORE

A 57-year-old woman:
— Presenting with irregular uterine bleeding

■ **Video 5.1**

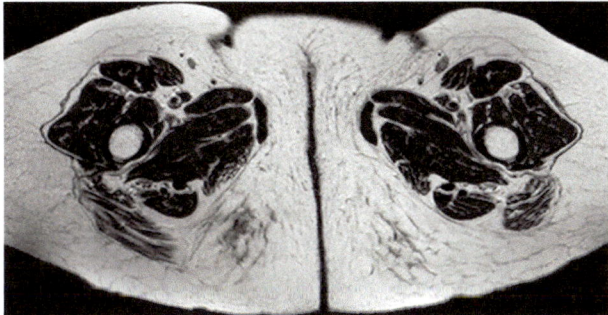

◻ Axial T2

5

■ **Video 5.2**

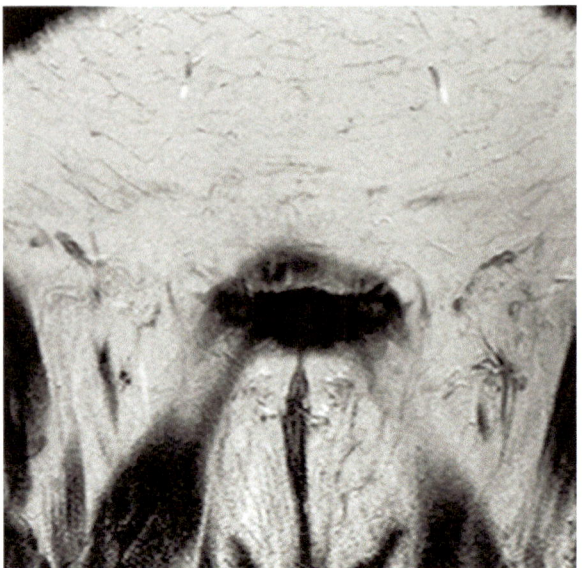

◘ Coronal T2

■ **Video 5.3**

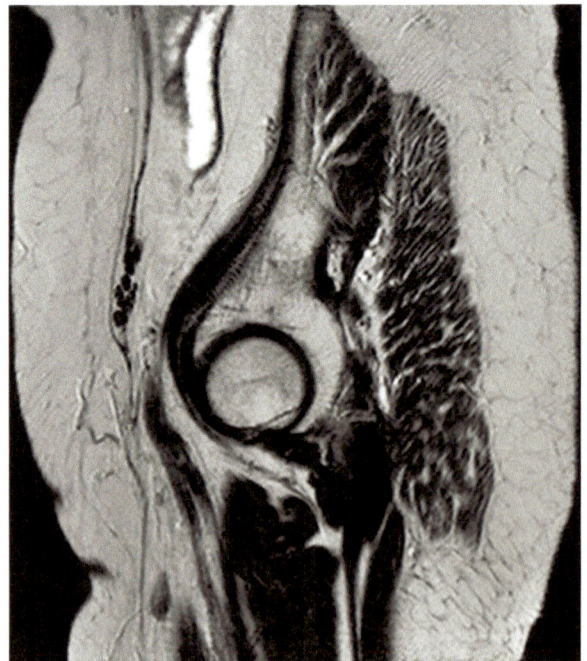

◘ Sagittal T2

Q1
Write down the three most relevant pelvic findings.

_____

_____

_____

 Q2

- **Video 5.4**

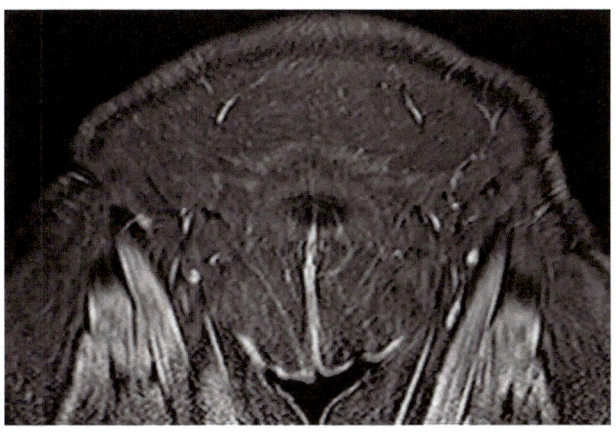

Which is the stage (FIGO 2009) of the disease?
(Only one option is correct.)
1. 1a
2. 1b
3. 2
4. 3b
5. 3c

 Q3
List the main imaging features to check for the staging of TNM endometrial carcinoma.

_____

_____

_____

Answers

Multiple Response Questions (MRQs)

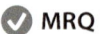 **MRQ 1**

2, 4 and 5

Explanation

The intrauterine contraceptive devices (IUCDs) are usually easily identified on standard two-dimensional (2D) transvaginal ultrasonography (TVUS) as linear echogenic structures (stem of IUCD) with various degree of visualisation of the arms. Three-dimensional (3D) US allows for a more detailed evaluation of the arm positioning. The possible complications of IUCD placement include uterine perforation, intraperitoneal migration, abscess or bowel injury. The risk of pelvic inflammatory disease (PID) is estimated to be threefold increased in patients with IUCD. The use of IUCDs is one of the risk factors of ectopic pregnancy.

MRQ 2

2

Explanation

Xanthogranulomatous pyelonephritis is an uncommon chronic renal infection diffusely affecting the kidney. On CT scans the kidney is enlarged with dilated calyces filled with hypoattenuating pus and reduced renal parenchyma. The renal pelvis is contracted and contains calculi. Perirenal inflammation is also easily depicted on CT as well as thickened perirenal fascia and fistulas.

MRQ 3

1, 3 and 4

Explanation

Differentiation of angiomyolipoma with minimal fat from renal cell carcinoma is difficult; biopsy or resection is necessary to attain the correct diagnosis.

The imaging findings of renal adenomas (hypovascular mass related to the normal renal parenchyma) often overlap with those of RCC.

Oncocytoma with good demarcation, spoke wheel pattern of contrast enhancement and central scar is not characteristic either, as these features may be seen in RCC as well.

Clear cell renal carcinomas constitute approximately 7% of all renal cancers. Papillary (10–15%) and chromophobe (<5%) renal cancers are much less frequent than clear cell carcinoma.

Lipid-poor angiomyolipomas constitute the minority of these lesions.

MRQ 4

A – Urethra

B – Vagina

C – Obturator internus muscle

D – Levator ani muscle

E – Anus

✅ MRQ 5

1, 3 and 5

✅ MRQ 6

5

✅ MRQ 7

1,4 and 5

Explanation

If in doubt, mother's life first, *and* in non-life-threatening situations and depending on availability, MRI may be an alternative to protect the foetus from radiation, *and* in potential life-threatening injuries, all mandatory X-ray and CT examinations are performed.

The indication check for radiological examinations will be made even more stringent, and special consideration will be given to whether it is possible to avoid methods without radiation exposure and to avoid the administration of contrast agents. Of course, in potentially life-threatening conditions of the mother, all necessary examinations are carried out, and in case of doubt, the mother's life is the first priority.

✅ MRQ 8

2, 3, 4, and 5

Explanation

Stranding around the ureter (swelling of the fat) may be useful in difficult cases, *and* if urolithiasis is apparent, CT is able to locate the problem region/height, *and* a low-dose CT protocol is recommended, *and* although unlikely, fornix rupture may be caused by intravenous contrast media application.

In most cases, ultrasound is only able to visualise concretions in the discharging urinary tract within the kidneys. However, the typical colic pain only occurs when a stone obstructs one of the three typical levels: (1) proximal ureter directly behind the renal pelvic outlet, (2) crossover with the iliac vessels and (3) bladder ostium (vesicoureteric junction). A native CT diagnosis below 1 mSv is sufficient to assess the stone size. Periureteral stranding may help in difficult cases and may also be of diagnostic value in cases when the stone has already passed into the bladder. In addition, dual-energy techniques allow a differentiation between calcium stones and uric acid stones, with the latter often treated by lytic medication.

Short Cases (SCs)

SC 1

✅ Q1

2

✅ Q2

2

Q3

5

 Q4

3

Explanation

Fibromuscular dysplasia is an idiopathic, segmentary, non-inflammatory and non-atherosclerotic disease that can affect all layers of small- and medium-calibre arteries. It represents 2–3% of arterial hypertension cases. Renal arteries are most often involved although the disease may affect any artery. It has a typical appearance of "string of beads" (small stenoses along a vessel with intervening areas of dilatation) and is found mainly in young women. Any kind of arteriography (MRA, CTA, DSA) will show the abnormalities, with MR angiography being the non-invasive method of choice. Angioplasty is a treatment method of choice with stent placement in selected cases ± medical therapy.

SC 2

 Q1

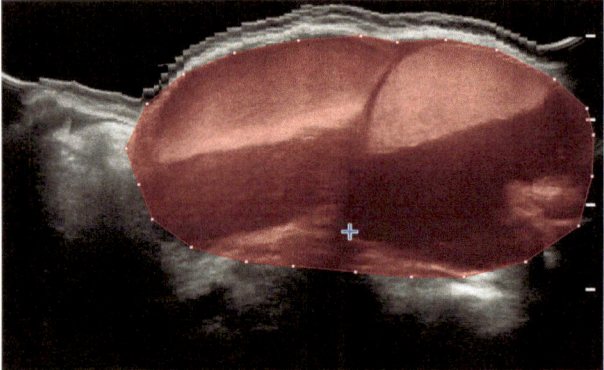

 Q2

4

 Q3

2, 4

 Q4

2

 Q5

2, 3 and 4

Explanation

Ovarian dermoid cysts or mature cystic teratomas (MCTs) are the most common ovarian neoplastic lesions in adolescents. They are benign germ cell tumours that arise from totipotent cells in the ovary which develop into fully differentiated ectodermal, mesodermal and endodermal tissue. They account for approximately 70% of benign ovarian tumours in females under 30 years of age and 50% of paediatric tumours. Ovarian dermoid cysts are usually asymptomatic and frequently are discovered incidentally. They are bilateral in approximately 10–20% of cases. Immature teratomas represent <1% of all ovarian teratomas and are also composed of tissue from the three germ cell layers; however, unlike MCTs, the cells are not fully differentiated.

SC 3
✔ **Q1**

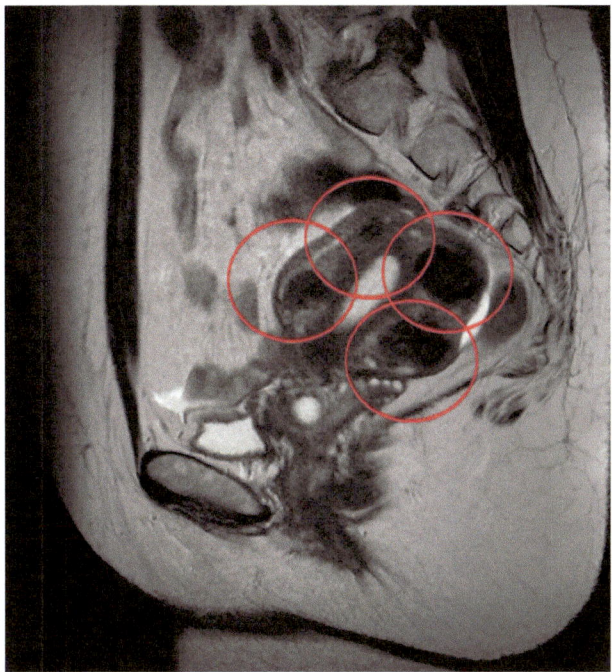

✔ **Q2**

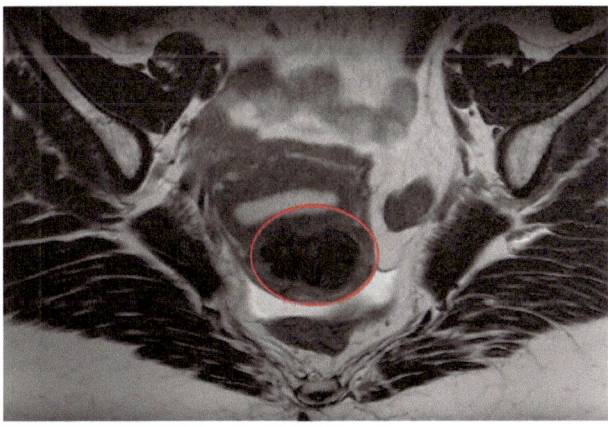

✅ **Q3**
1, 2, 3 and 5

✅ **Q4**
3 and 5

✅ **Q5**
Uterine fibroids; myomas OR leiomyomas.

CORE

5

✅ **Q1**
1. A lesion is detected at the body fundus of uterus with defined margins that show intermediate signal intensity in T2WI and is hyperintense compared with the myometrium. The mass is confined to uterus, distends the endometrial cavity, compresses the myometrium and involves more than 50% of the myometrial thickness. No cervical stromal invasion or extrauterine spread neither lymphadenopathies are detected. These findings are consistent with endometrial cancer stage Ib (FIGO MRI assessment).
2. In the posterior uterine wall, at the level of the fundus, an intramural lesion is identified with low signal intensity in T2WI, consistent with uterine leiomyoma.
3. The uterus is retroverted and retroflexed.
4. The left ovary shows a follicle.

✅ **Q2**
2

✅ **Q3**
– *Extension within the uterus*:
   (To determine the depth of myometrial invasion, a line is drawn parallel to the presumed inner edge of the myometrium. Then, two perpendicular lines are drawn: one measures the thickness of the entire myometrium, and the other measures the maximum tumour extent into the myometrium. The ratio of the lengths equals the depth of myometrial invasion.)
   – IA: Tumour confined to uterus, with less than 50% of myometrial thickness involvement
   – IB: Tumour confined to uterus, with more than 50% of myometrial thickness involvement
– *Cervical stroma invasion (stage II)*:
   Tumour invades the cervical stroma but does not extend beyond the uterus. Cervical stromal invasion is detected by the disruption or focal thinning of cervical stroma, and it is best assessed by evaluating both the sagittal and axial oblique planes that are acquired parallel and perpendicular to the long axis of the cervix, respectively.

— *Tumour extension:*
  - IIIA: Uterine serosa invasion or direct tumour spread to the adnexa or ovarian metastases
  - IIIB: Invasion of the vagina or parametrium by either direct invasion or metastatic spread
  - IIIC: Presence of lymph node metastases. This stage is subdivided on the basis of pelvic (stage IIIC1) and/or para-aortic (stage IIIC2) lymph node involvement
  - IV: Direct invasion of the bladder or rectal mucosa (stage IVA) or distant metastases (stage IVB). The assessment is largely based on size criteria where a short axis diameter of greater than 8 mm in pelvic nodes and 10 mm in para-aortic nodes is taken to indicate tumoural involvement

Literature

Andreano A, Rechichi G, Rebora P, Sironi S, Valsecchi MG, Galimberti S. MR diffusion imaging for preoperative staging of myometrial invasion in patients with endometrial cancer: a systematic review and meta-analysis. Eur Radiol. 2014;24(6):1327–38.

Bonatti M, Lombardo F, Vezzali N, et al. MDCT of blunt renal trauma: imaging findings and therapeutic implications. Insights into Imaging. 2015;6(2):261–72.

Hosseinzadeh K, Heller MT, Houshmand G. Imaging of the female perineum in adults. Radiographics. 2012;32:129–68.

Kinkel K, Forstner R, Danza FM, et al. Staging of endometrial cancer with MRI: guidelines of the European Society of Urogenital Imaging. Eur Radiol. 2009;19(7):1565–74.

Nougaret S, Horta M, Lakhman Y, et al. Endometrial cancer MRI staging: updated guidelines of the European Society of Urogenital Radiology. Eur Radiol. Available via https://www.ncbi.nlm.nih.gov/pubmed/2999523920. Accessed 18 July 2018.

Rechichi G, Galimberti S, Signorelli M, Perego P, Valsecchi MG, Sironi S. Myometrial invasion in endometrial cancer: diagnostic performance of diffusion-weighted MR imaging at 1.5-T. Eur Radiol. 2010;20(3):754–62.

Tirkes T, Sandrasegaran K, Patel AA, Hollar MA, et al. Peritoneal and retroperitoneal anatomy and its relevance for cross-sectional imaging. Radiographics. 2012;32:437–51.

Wasnik AP, Mazza MB, Liu PS. Normal and variant pelvic anatomy on MRI. Magn Reson Imaging Clin N Am. 2011;19(3):547–66.

Additional EDiR Preparatory Materials

http://learn.myesr.org

EDiR Preparatory Sessions

http://learn.myesr.org
Staging of prostate cancer.
Imaging evaluation of the indeterminate adrenal mass.
Imaging of gynaecological malignancies.

Head and Neck Radiology

Electronic supplementary material   The online version of this chapter
(https://doi.org/10.1007/978-3-030-20066-4_6) contains supplementary material,
which is available to authorized users.

Multiple Response Questions (MRQs)

❓ MRQ 1

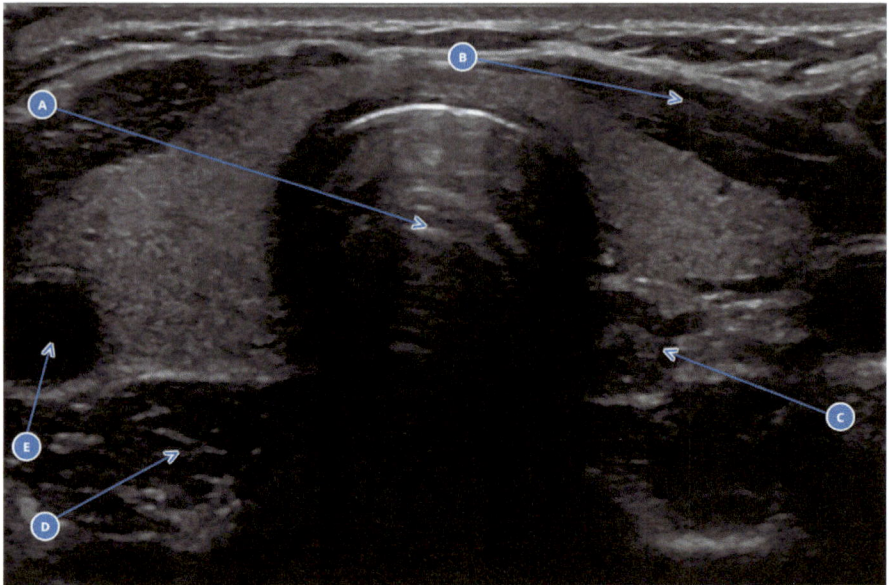

Associate the labels with the following list of structures.
1. Trachea
2. Longus colli muscle
3. Sternohyoid muscle
4. Common carotid artery
5. Jugular vein
6. Oesophagus

❓ MRQ 2
What are the CT findings of right vocal cord paralysis?
(Multiple answers might be correct.)
1. Posterolateral rotation of the left arytenoid cartilage
2. Fatty infiltration of the right vocal cord
3. Ballooning of the left laryngeal ventricle
4. Medial deviation of right aryepiglottic fold
5. Enlarged left pyriform sinus

❓ MRQ 3

When is the usual time to perform a baseline MRI/CT after chemo-/radiation therapy in head and neck tumours?

(Only one answer is correct.)

1. 1 week
2. 1 month
3. 3 months
4. 6 months
5. 1 year

❓ MRQ 4

Regarding juvenile angiofibromas, which statement is correct?

(Multiple answers might be correct.)

1. They arise at the sphenopalatine foramen
2. They typically cause widening of the pterygopalatine fossa
3. They are benign tumours
4. They occur most frequently in adolescent females
5. They are supplied by the internal maxillary artery

Short Cases (SCs)

SC 1

A 45-year-old male:

▬ Chronic diffuse neck pain increased over several years

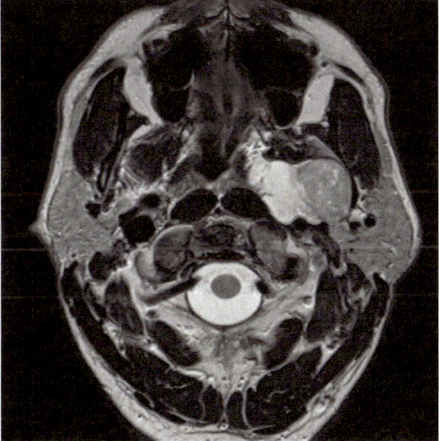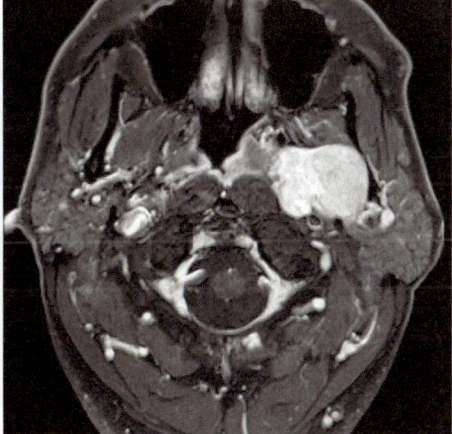

? Q1

Where do you think the abnormality seen on the images is arising from?

_____

_____

_____

? Q2

What is the most likely diagnosis?
(Only one option is correct.)
1. Schwannoma of the vagus nerve
2. Parapharyngeal space branchial cleft cyst
3. Pleomorphic adenoma of the parotid gland
4. Rhabdomyoma of the perivertebral space
5. Parapharyngeal space hemangioma

? Q3

Which of the following procedures would you recommend?
(Only one option is correct.)
1. Fine-needle aspiration
2. PET-CT
3. Ultrasound
4. Surgical removal
5. Wait and see

? Q4

Which of the following complications might be seen in this patient?
(Only one answer is correct.)
1. Infection
2. Malignant degeneration
3. None
4. Meningitis
5. Spontaneous bleeding

SC 2

Male with rapid progressive neck swelling and dyspnoea:

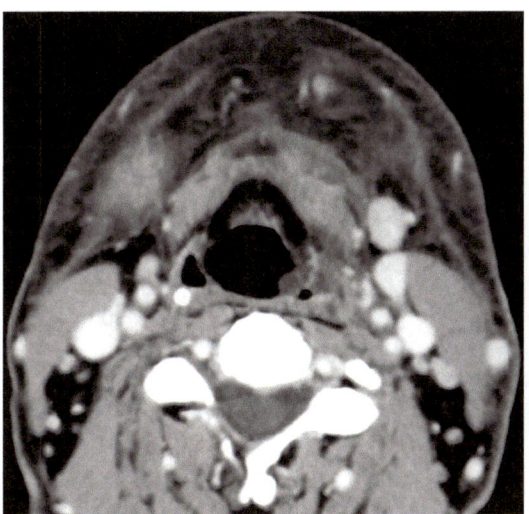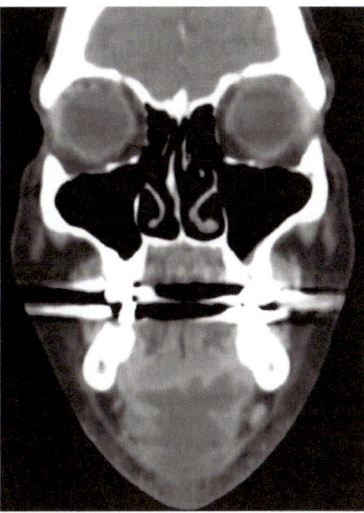

❓ Q1

What radiological features do you recognise in the images?

(Multiple answers might be correct.)

1. Necrotic lymphadenopathy
2. Floor of the mouth abscess
3. Anterior neck abscess
4. Myositis paravertebral muscles
5. Anterior neck cellulitis

❓ Q2

Which of the following would you include in the differential diagnosis?

(Multiple answers might be correct.)

1. Suppurative lymphadenitis
2. Cellulitis of the floor of the mouth (Ludwig's angina)
3. Necrotising fasciitis
4. Phlegmon
5. Erysipelas

? Q3

What course of actions would you take next?

(Multiple answers might be correct.)

1. MRI for further diagnosis
2. Immediate surgery
3. Fine-needle aspiration
4. Oral antibiotics and follow-up CT
5. Intravenous antibiotics

? Q4

Which of the following statements regarding necrotising fasciitis are correct?

(Multiple answers might be correct.)

1. Immediate surgery is of upmost importance
2. Absence of air within the soft tissues on CT excludes necrotising fasciitis
3. Involvement of the platysma and anterior neck is characteristic
4. Typical multiple neck compartments are involved
5. The mediastinum and the lung are rarely involved at initial presentation

CORE

A 64-year-old man:

- With a history of smoking (40 packs/year)
- Presented with a left neck swelling and left ear pain

- **Video 6.1**

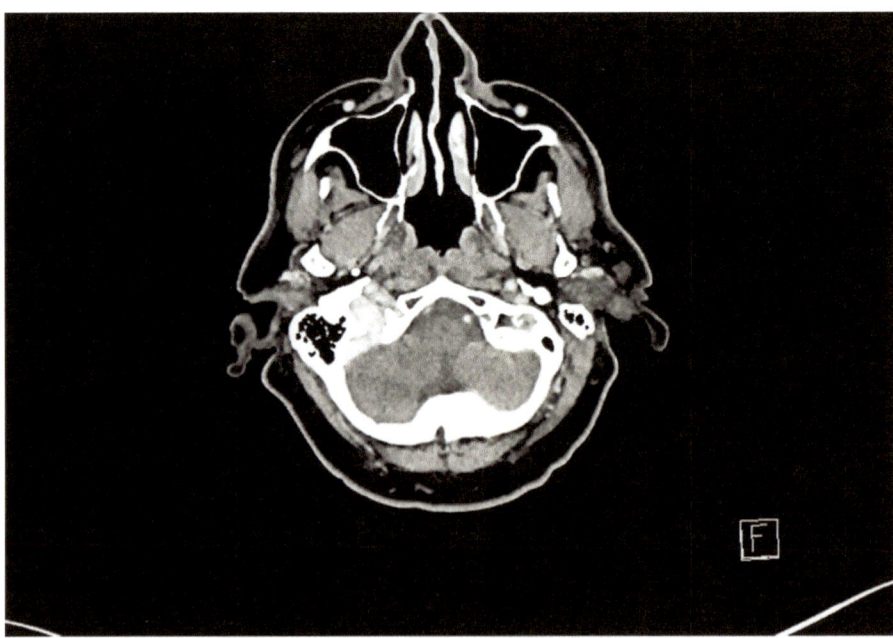

❓ Q1

What is the location of the primary lesion in this patient?

(Choose one of the following options.)

1. Left tonsil
2. Base of the tongue
3. Oral cavity
4. Prevertebral space
5. Carotid space

❓ Q2

What is the most likely diagnosis of the lesions that is causing the left neck swelling?

(Choose one of the following options.)

1. Left lymph node
2. Left schwannoma
3. Left jugular vein thrombosis
4. Left carotid dissection
5. Left parotid pleomorphic adenoma

❓ Q3

Which characteristics are indicative of a pathological lymph node?

(Multiple answers might be correct.)

1. Increased size
2. Presence of necrosis
3. Fatty hilum
4. Extranodal extension
5. Decreased vascularity on ultrasound

❓ Q4

In which level is the enlarged left-sided lymph node of this patient located?

_____

_____

_____

❓ Q5

In which anatomical region is the primary lesion of this patient located?

(Only one option is correct.)

1. Oropharynx
2. Oral cavity
3. Nasopharynx
4. Retropharyngeal space
5. Hypopharynx

? **Q6**

Why is the patient experiencing left ear pain?

(Only one option is correct.)

1. Perineural tumour spread
2. Referred pain
3. External otitis
4. Acute tonsillitis
5. Mastoiditis

Answers

Multiple Response Questions (MRQs)

6

✓ **MRQ 1**

1A, 2D, 3B, 4E, 5 (not seen) and 6C

✓ **MRQ 2**

2 and 4

✓ **MRQ 3**

3

Explanation

Within the first 2 weeks after radiotherapy, there is an acute inflammatory reaction within the deep tissues. Irradiation produces tissue changes on post-treatment imaging studies that should not be misinterpreted as evidence of persistent or recurrent disease. A baseline study is recommended 3 months after the end of therapy.

✓ **MRQ 4**

1, 2, 3 and 5

Explanation

Juvenile nasopharyngeal angiofibroma is a highly vascular neoplasm that tends to spread in the various fissures and foramina of the nasopharynx; they are more frequently found in young male adolescents.

Short Cases (SCs)

SC 1

 Q1

Left deep parotid lobe. The tumour arises from the deep lobe of the parotid. They classically appear as well-defined, multilobulated T2 hyperintense tumors with heterogeneous nodular enhancement.

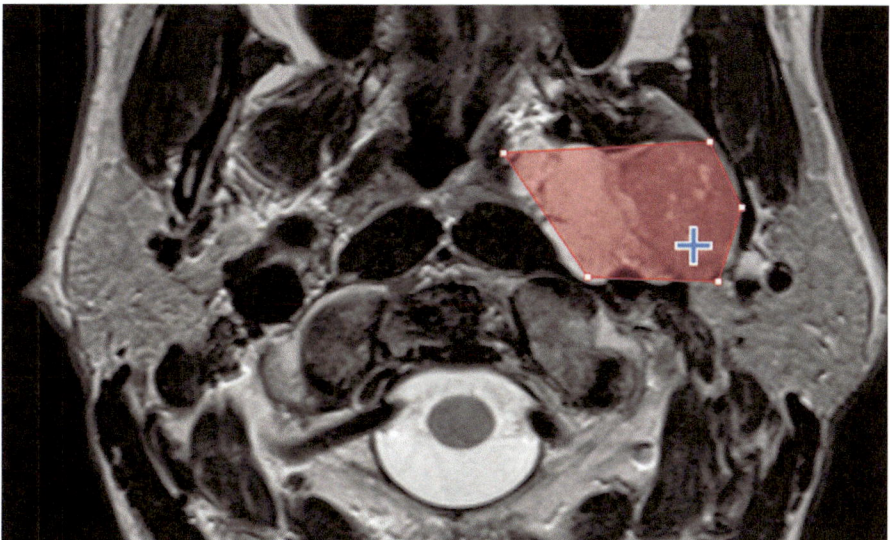

 Q2

Pleomorphic adenoma
Explanation
Pleomorphic adenomas are the most common tumours of the parotid gland.

 Q3

4

 Q4

2
Explanation
Pleomorphic adenomas are benign tumours; however, long-standing lesions can have malignant degeneration. Carcinoma ex pleomorphic adenoma is a very aggressive tumour with a poor prognosis. Therefore, all pleomorphic adenomas should be removed surgically. Differential diagnosis includes schwannoma, haemangioma and lymph node.

SC 2

✅ **Q1**
2 and 5

✅ **Q2**
2 and 3

✅ **Q3**
2 and 5

✅ **Q4**
1, 3 and 4
Explanation
Necrotising fasciitis is a bacterial life-threatening infection of the face/neck with fulminant clinical evolution. Mortality: 15–70%. Causes: odontogenic, tonsillar and pharyngeal infection. Treatment: surgery+antibiotics+airway support.

CORE

✅ **Q1**
1

✅ **Q2**
1

✅ **Q3**
1, 2 and 4
Explanation
Most nodes in the head and neck should be <10 mm in short axis except:
Submental/submandibular and jugulodigastric <15 mm
Retropharyngeal <8 mm.

✅ **Q4**
IIA
Explanation
Level IIA: anterior, lateral, medial or posterior to the internal jugular vein. If the node is posterior to the internal jugular vein, it must be inseparable from it.

✅ **Q5**
1

✅ **Q6**
2
Explanation
The glossopharyngeal nerve (CN IX), when involved by oropharyngeal cancers (tonsil, base of tongue), can cause referred ear pain.

Literature

Bin Saeedan M, Aljohani IM, Khushaim AO, Bukhari SQ, Elnaas ST. Thyroid computed tomography imaging: pictorial review of variable pathologies. Insights Imaging. 2016;7:601–17.

Dankbaar JW, Pameijer FA. Vocal cord paralysis: anatomy, imaging and pathology. Insights Imaging. 2014;5:743–51.

Dankbaar JW, van Bemmel AJ, Pameijer FA. Imaging findings of the orbital and intracranial complications of acute bacterial rhinosinusitis. Insights Imaging. 2015;6:509–18.

Patel S, Bhatt AA. Imaging of the sublingual and submandibular spaces. Insights Imaging. 2018;9(3): 391–401.

Purohit BS, Ailianou A, Dulguerov N, et al. FDG-PET/CT pitfalls in oncological head and neck imaging. Insights Imaging. 2014;5:585–602.

Purohit BS, Vargas MI, Ailianou A, et al. Orbital tumours and tumour-like lesions: exploring the armamentarium of multiparametric imaging. Insights Imaging. 2016;7:43–68.

Tashi S, Purohit BS, Becker M, Mundada P. The pterygopalatine fossa: imaging anatomy, communications, and pathology revisited. Insights Imaging. 2016;7:589–99.

Additional EDiR Preparatory Materials

http://learn.myesr.org

EDiR Preparatory Sessions

http://learn.myesr.org
Oral cavity and oropharyngeal pathology.
Laryngeal and hypopharyngeal pathology.
Neck lymph nodes.

Interventional and Vascular Radiology

© European Board of Radiology (EBR) 2019
J. Babar et al., *EDiR - The Essential Guide*, https://doi.org/10.1007/978-3-030-20066-4_7

Multiple Response Questions (MRQs)

❓ MRQ 1
CT images of haemodynamically stable patient after blunt abdominal trauma:

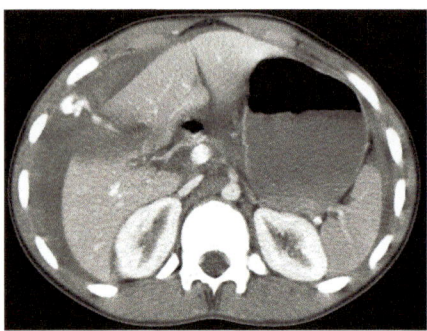 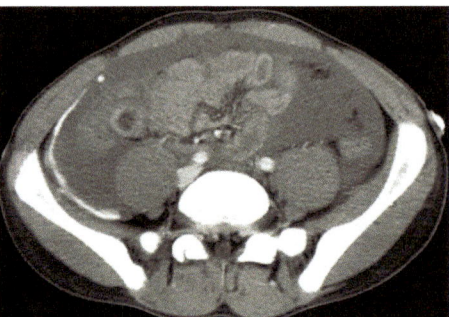

Which of the following statements are correct regarding these images?
(Multiple answers might be correct.)
1. There is haemoperitoneum
2. There is evidence of active bleeding
3. Angiography and embolisation are indicated in this patient
4. Embolisation for traumatic bleeding is preferably performed with embolisation particles
5. The patient should be referred immediately to surgery

❓ MRQ 2
Which of the following are commonly recognised risk factors in postpartum haemorrhage?
(Multiple answers might be correct.)
1. Pre-existing bleeding disorders
2. Multiple pregnancies
3. Hydramnios
4. Previous postpartum haemorrhage
5. Chinese ethnic origin

❓ MRQ 3
Which of the following statements are correct regarding endoleaks following endovascular abdominal aortic aneurysm repair?
(Multiple answers might be correct.)
1. Type III endoleaks result from modular disconnection
2. Type 1 endoleak is the most frequently encountered endoleak
3. Type I and type III endoleaks are the most commonly associated in rupture of the aneurysm sac
4. Type II endoleak is caused by a tear in the fabric of the graft material
5. The incidence of type I endoleak increases over 12 months

❓ MRQ 4

A 67-year-old man presents with abdominal pain and vomiting and undergoes a contrast-enhanced CT scan:

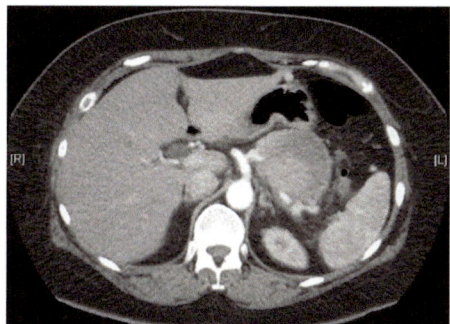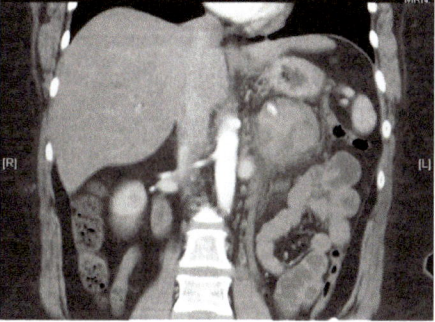

Which of the following statements are correct?
(Multiple answers might be correct.)

1. There is a large splenic artery aneurysm
2. There is a large pseudocyst in the tail of pancreas
3. There is a large gastrointestinal stromal tumour (GIST)
4. The optimal treatment is surgical resection
5. Radiofrequency ablation will result in cure in 35% of patients if no additional lesion is seen on the CT scan

❓ MRQ 5

Which of the following is an exclusion criterion for radioembolisation of a liver tumour?
(Only one option is correct.)

1. Splenorenal shunt
2. Significant hepatopulmonary shunting
3. Minor tumoural arterioportal shunting
4. Aberrant hepatic artery
5. Occlusion of the gastroduodenal artery

Short Cases (SCs)

SC 1

A 70-year-old female patient with a history of smoking and hypertension:
— The patient presents with chest and abdominal pain

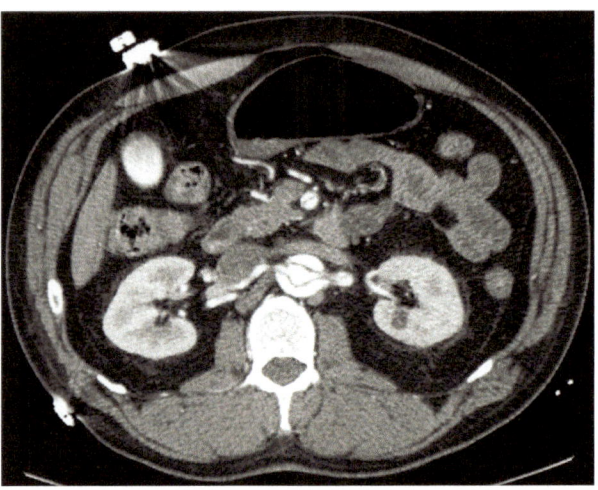

❓ Q1
Which is the most likely diagnosis?
(Only one answer is correct.)
1. Intramural haematoma
2. Aortic stenosis
3. Penetrating aortic ulcer
4. Abdominal aortic aneurysm
5. Aortic dissection

❓ Q2
The dissection starts from just distal to the subclavian artery, and the patient has high blood pressure but is otherwise stable. What are the best treatment options?
(Multiple answers might be correct.)
1. Review with repeat CT scan at intervals and correlate with clinical symptoms
2. Anticoagulate the patient
3. Immediately place a stent-graft
4. Plan elective open surgery when blood pressure is controlled
5. Medical therapy for blood pressure control

Answers

Multiple Response Questions (MRQs)

✅ MRQ 1

1, 2 and 3

✅ MRQ 2

1, 2, 3 and 4

Explanation

According to the WHO, obstetric haemorrhage affects around 10% of all live births and accounts for 24% of maternal deaths worldwide. In developed countries, it is estimated there are 9–17 maternal deaths per 10,000 deliveries related to postpartum haemorrhage (PPH), as compared to 400 death per 10,000 deliveries worldwide.

Several studies emphasize the statistically significant increased odds of atonic postpartum hemorrhage in Asian ethnic origin. The most common cause of PPH is uterine atony, when the normal myometrium fails to contract after delivery of the placenta. Other common causes include genital or vaginal lacerations, abnormal placentation, multiple pregnancies, hydramnios, AVMs, pseudoaneurysms, congenital or acquired coagulation disorders, uterine rupture or inversion.

✅ MRQ 3

1, 3 and 5

Explanation

Type I endoleaks (EL) are defined as a leak at the attachment site of an endograft and a manifestation of sealing failure. Type I EL are further subclassified into types IA, IB and IC depending on the occurrence at proximal and distal end of the endograft, or iliac occluder, respectively.

Type II EL are branch endoleaks and involve retrograde flow into the aneurysm sac from aortic or iliac branch arteries, such as intercostal, lumbar, inferior mesenteric and hypogastric arteries. They are further differentiated into type IIA when they are related to only one patent branch and type IIB when they are complex with two or more patent branches and creating a flow-through situation.

Type III EL are defined as a junctional leaks, modular disconnection (IIIA) or fabric disruption with midgraft holes (IIIB).

Type IV EL are defined as a porous endograft, which is detected 30 days after graft placement, due to fabric porosity. By definition, an endoleak noted on follow-up imaging should not be considered as type IV endoleak.

Type V EL refer to the phenomenon of endotension, which represents a persistent or recurrent pressurisation of an aneurysm sac without an identifiable type I–IV endoleaks on imaging.

✅ MRQ 4

1

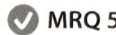 **MRQ 5**

2

Explanation

The absolute contraindications to radioembolisation for any malignancy include severely compromised hepatic function, poor performance status (ECOG 4 2), active hepatic infection, significant extrahepatic metastases and pregnancy. After mapping angiography, the inability to administer ^{90}Y microspheres without nontarget embolisation to the bowel is also considered as an absolute contraindication. A high lung shunt fraction (LSF) that would lead to a greater than 30-Gy dose to the lungs with a single treatment is an absolute contraindication for radioembolisation. Relative contraindications to radioembolisation include uncorrectable coagulopathy, severe radiographic contrast medium allergy and renal impairment, all of which can often be medically addressed. Increased bilirubin level and significant ascites are relative contraindications; individualised patient decision-making is recommended in these settings.

7

Short Cases (SCs)

SC 1

 Q1

5

 Q2

1 and 5

Explanation

Medical management with anti-impulse therapy has remained the preferred treatment option for uncomplicated acute type B dissection, with in-hospital mortality rates typically <10% with this strategy. Long-term mortality after hospital discharge is greater for type B dissection than for type A dissection, and attentive medical management and aortic surveillance are required. Specific predictors of follow-up mortality include female gender, prior aortic aneurysm, atherosclerosis, pleural effusion and in-hospital acute renal failure, hypotension or shock. Medical management with β-blockade and blood pressure control remains the cornerstone of long-term therapy for type B dissection; however, a recent report from IRAD also found that the use of calcium channel blockers at discharge was associated with improved long-term survival selectively in medically treated type B dissection patients.

Literature

Choo SJ. Treatment of uncomplicated acute type B aortic dissection in the endovascular era: is it time for a paradigm shift? J Thorac Dis. 2017;9(10):3450–2.

Corvera JS. Acute aortic syndrome. Ann Cardiothorac Surg. 2016;5(3):188–93.

Etesami M, Ashwath R, Kanne J, Gilkeson RC, Rajiah P. Computed tomography in the evaluation of vascular rings and slings. Insights into Imaging. 2014;5:507–21.

Gonsalves M, Belli A. The role of interventional radiology in obstetric hemorrhage. Cardiovasc Intervent Radiol. 2010;33(5):887–95.

Mauri G, Mattiuz C, Sconfienza LM, et al. Role of interventional radiology in the management of complications after pancreatic surgery: a pictorial review. Insights into Imaging. 2015;6:231–9.

Murphy DJ, Aghayev A, Steigner ML. Vascular CT and MRI: a practical guide to imaging protocols. Insights into Imaging. 2018;9(2):215–36.

Padia SA, Lewandowski RJ, Johnson GE, et al., for the Society of Interventional Radiology Standards of Practice Committee. Radioembolization of hepatic malignancies: background, quality improvement guidelines, and future directions. J Vasc Interv Radiol. 2017;28(1):1–15.

Rand T, Uberoi R, Cil B, Munneke G, Tsetis D. Quality improvement guidelines for imaging detection and treatment of Endoleaks following endovascular aneurysm repair (EVAR). Cardiovasc Intervent Radiol. 2013;36:35–45.

Additional EDiR Preparatory Materials

http://learn.myesr.org

EDiR Preparation Sessions

http://learn.myesr.org
Basic principles of angiography and image-guided interventions.
Vascular interventions.
Interventions of the hepatobiliary system.

Musculoskeletal Radiology

Electronic supplementary material   The online version of this chapter (https://doi.org/10.1007/978-3-030-20066-4_8) contains supplementary material, which is available to authorized users.

Multiple Response Questions (MRQs)

❓ MRQ 1

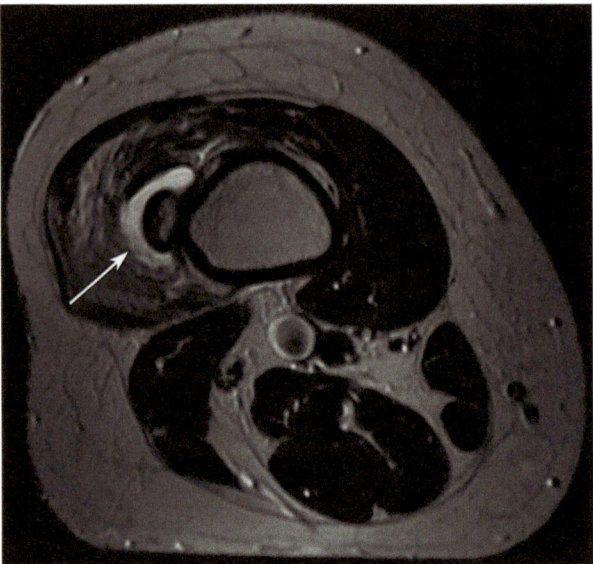

Which of the following statements are correct regarding this image?
(Multiple answers might be correct.)
1. There is an increased risk of malignancy in this condition
2. Normal/normal variant
3. This could be a sign of an autosomal dominant disorder
4. This condition is rarely seen in the long tubular bones
5. The lesions, as pointed out by the arrow, are always solitary

❓ MRQ 2
Which of the following conditions can cause unilateral protrusio acetabuli?
(Multiple answers might be correct.)
1. Rheumatoid arthritis
2. Paget's disease
3. Diabetes
4. Tuberculous arthritis
5. Fibrous dysplasia

8

? MRQ 3

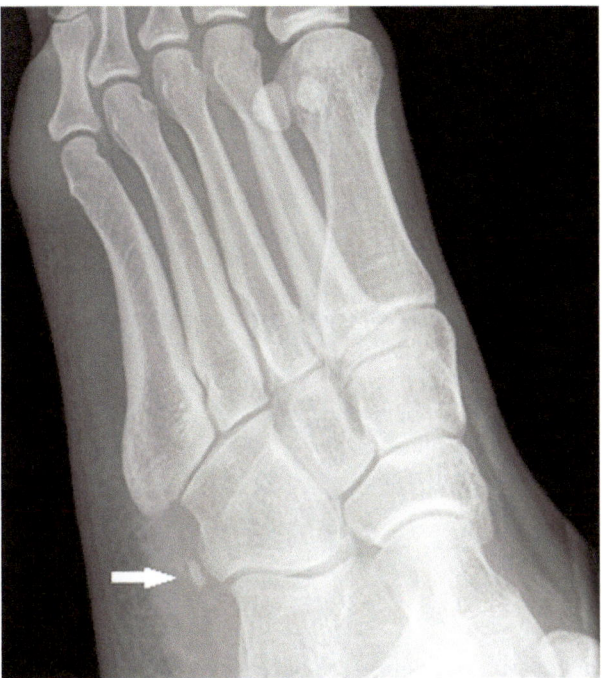

Which of the following statements are correct regarding this image?
(Multiple answers might be correct.)
1. There is an avulsion fracture
2. This condition may be caused by trauma
3. This condition is normal/normal variant
4. This appearance is commonly seen bilaterally
5. This finding can cause peroneus longus tenosynovitis

? MRQ 4
Regarding transient patellar dislocation (TPD), which of the following statements are correct?
(Multiple answers might be correct.)
1. Bone oedema following TPD classically affects the lateral patellar facet and medial femoral condyle
2. Normal trochlear depth is > 5 mm
3. Risk is increased by patella baja deformity
4. TPD is frequently associated with tears of the medial collateral ligament
5. Tibial Tuberosity–Trochlear groove distance (TT–TG) < 16 mm is normal

❓ MRQ 5

Regarding gout, which of the following statements are correct?

(Multiple answers might be correct.)

1. Bony erosions demonstrate sclerotic borders
2. Mineralisation of bone is typically decreased
3. Bony erosions with overhanging edges are typical in gout
4. Tophaceous deposition can occur in tendons
5. Chondrocalcinosis is generally present in gout

❓ MRQ 6

Regarding musculoskeletal manifestations of scleroderma, which of the following imaging signs are correct?

(Multiple answers might be correct.)

1. The hands are the most common site of involvement
2. Subcutaneous and periarticular calcification
3. Resorption of the first carpometacarpal joint
4. Sclerosis of the rib and mandibular angle
5. Hypertrophy of the tip of the fingers

❓ MRQ 7

Which of the following radiographic findings are seen in primary hyperparathyroidism?

(Multiple answers might be correct.)

1. Mixed osteopenia and osteosclerosis
2. Soft tissue calcification
3. Subperiosteal bone resorption
4. Subchondral resorption
5. Chondrocalcinosis

❓ MRQ 8

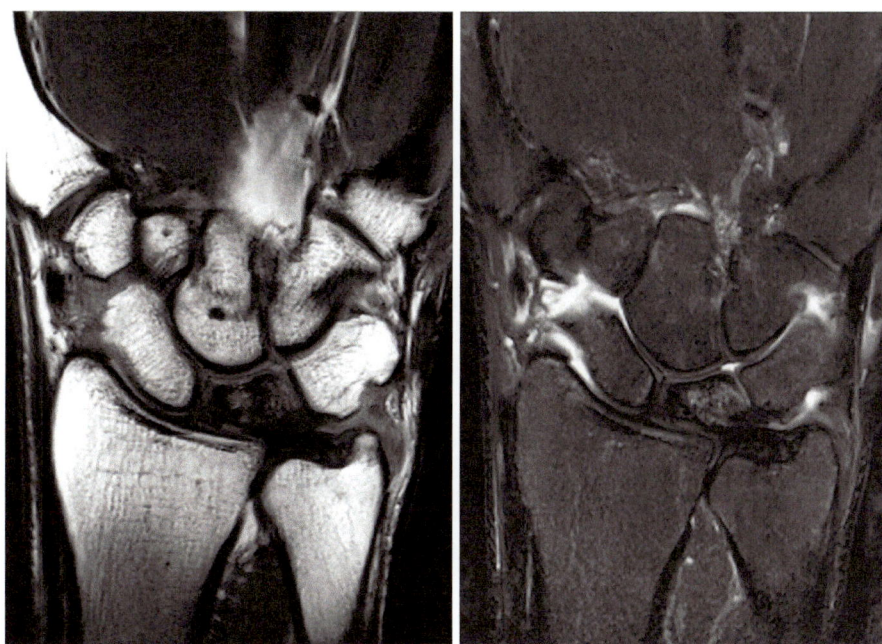

Regarding this patient with chronic wrist pain, which of the following statements are correct?

(Multiple answers might be correct.)

1. Chronic repetitive trauma is a risk factor
2. Vascularised bone grafting is a treatment option
3. There is high T1 signal intensity of the lunate
4. There is a scaphoid fracture
5. This entity is typically associated with positive ulnar variance

❓ MRQ 9

Regarding osteosarcoma of the long bones, which of the following statements are correct?

(Multiple answers might be correct.)

1. It is the most common primary malignant tumour of bone in adolescence
2. A lamellated periosteal reaction is never seen
3. Para-osteal variant of osteosarcoma shows more aggressive features than other subtypes
4. The epiphysis is the commonest site in the bones around the knee
5. A characteristic feature is calcification of the tumour matrix

Short Cases (SCs)

SC 1

A 23-year-old male:
- Known epileptic
- Following a seizure presents with shoulder pain and restricted shoulder movement
- X-ray is performed

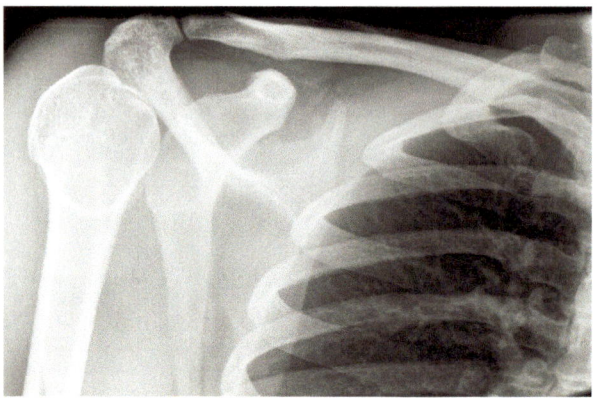

❓ Q1
What does the radiography demonstrate?
(Multiple answers might be correct.)
1. Internal rotation of the humeral head resulting in the light bulb sign
2. Detached anteroinferior labrum and avulsion fracture of the glenoid rim—bony Bankart
3. Overlap of the humeral head and impaction fracture resulting in the trough sign
4. Normal appearances
5. Fracture of the posterior aspect of the humeral head—A Hill–Sachs lesion

❓ Q2
Which is the most likely diagnosis?
(Only one answer is correct.)
1. Anterior glenohumeral joint dislocation
2. Posterior glenohumeral joint dislocation
3. Lesser tuberosity fracture
4. Acromioclavicular disruption
5. Greater tuberosity fracture

❓ Q3

What injuries are associated with this condition?
(Multiple answers might be correct.)

1. Reverse Bankart lesion
2. Bankart lesion
3. Reverse Hill–Sachs lesion
4. Fracture of the lesser tuberosity
5. Hill–Sachs lesion

❓ Q4

Four years later, the patient presents in orthopaedic clinic with shoulder instability. A shoulder arthrogram is performed.

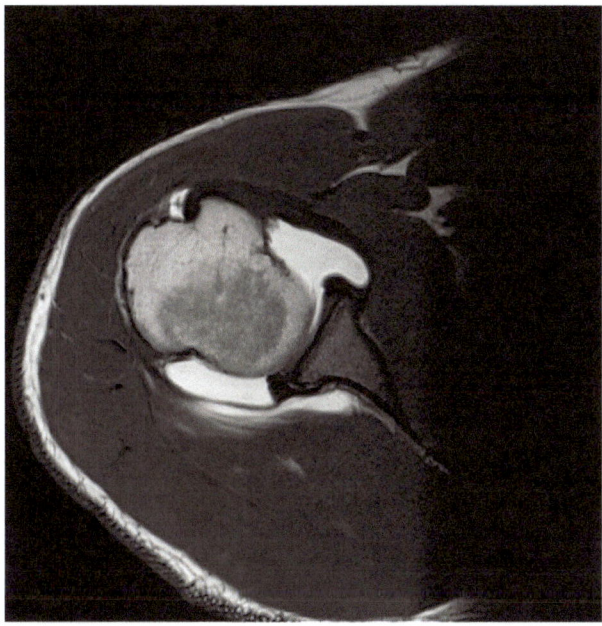

What does the arthrogram confirm?

_____

_____

_____

SC 2

A 41-year-old female patient:

— The patient presented with slowly growing swelling at the base of the right great toe for 2 months

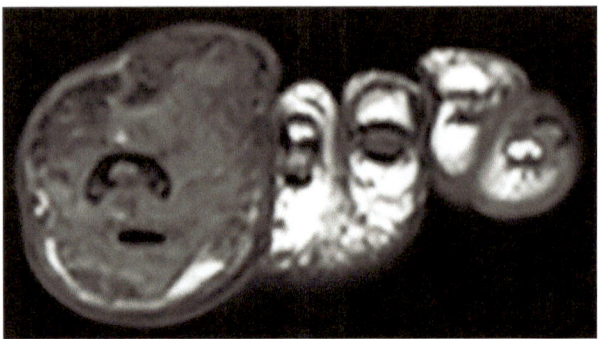

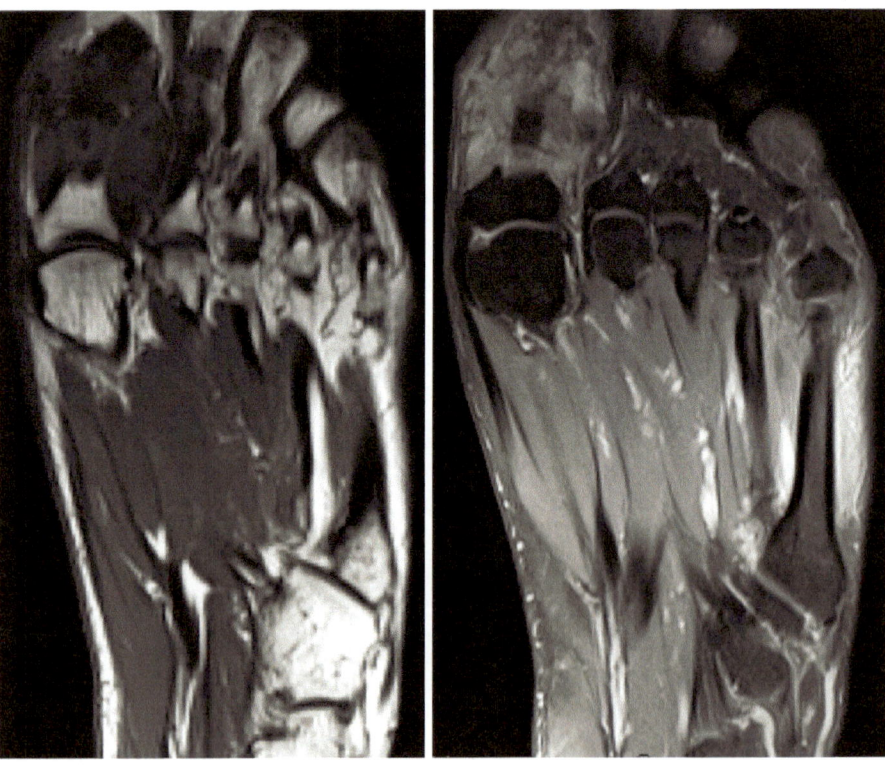

❓ Q1
Indicate the abnormality.

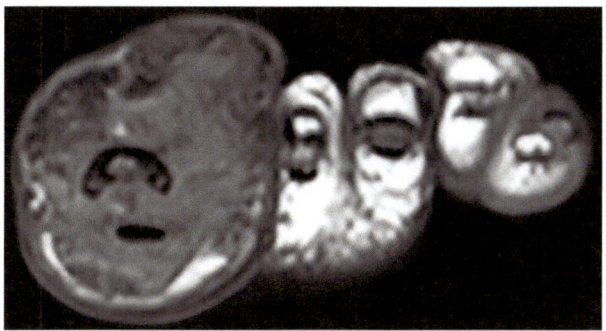

❓ Q2
The patient was referred for an ultrasound-guided biopsy of the lesion, differential diagnosis includes:
(Multiple answers might be correct.)
1. Desmoid tumour
2. Giant cell tumour of the tendon sheath/pigmented villonodular synovitis
3. Morton's neuroma
4. Glomus tumour
5. Infection

❓ Q3
What is the most likely diagnosis?
(Only one option is correct.)
1. Vascular malformation
2. Giant cell tumour of the tendon sheath/pigmented villonodular synovitis
3. Infection
4. Morton's neuroma
5. Gout

❓ Q4
What are the imaging features of giant cell tumours of the tendon sheath on MRI?
(Multiple answers might be correct.)
1. Low T1-weighted and T2-weighted signal intensity
2. Low T1-weighted and high T2-weighted signal intensity
3. Low signal intensity on gradient echo and may demonstrate blooming
4. High T1-weighted and T2-weighted signal intensity
5. Might demonstrate enhancement post-intravenous contrast administration

SC 3

A 56-year-old gentleman:
- Presents with 2-week history of worsening back pain
- No radiculopathy
- Previously fit and well

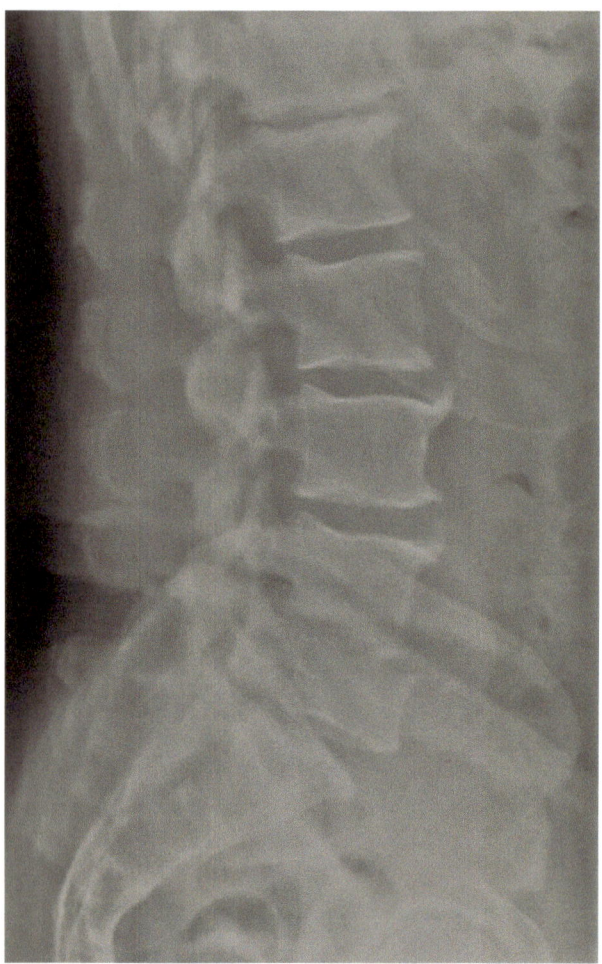

❓ Q1
Indicate the abnormality.

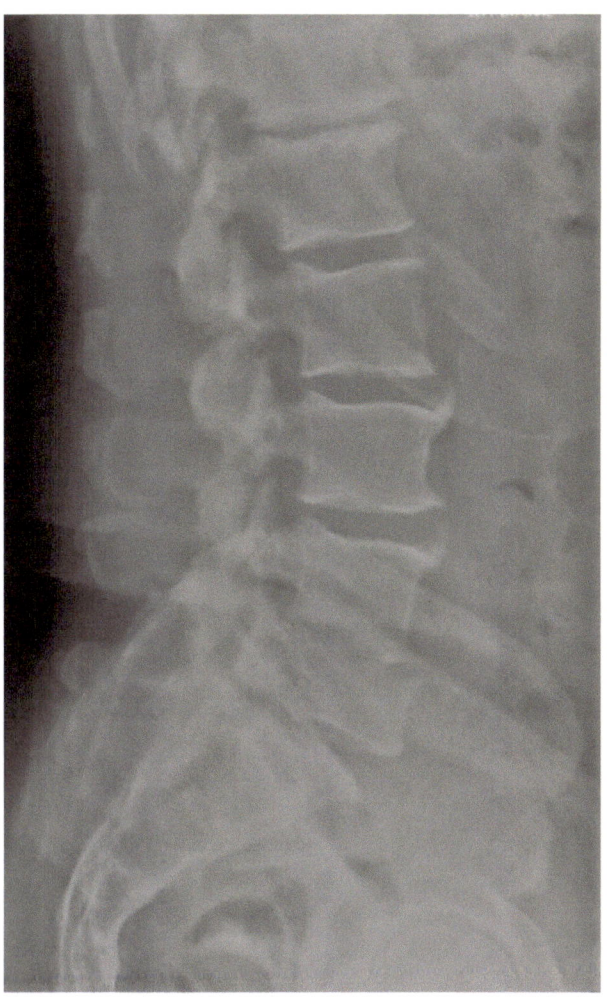

❓ Q2
What differential diagnosis should be considered in an inflammatory discovertebral lesion?
(Multiple answers might be correct.)
1. Modic type III changes
2. Spondylodiscitis
3. Gout
4. Ankylosing spondylitis
5. Diffuse idiopathic skeletal hyperostosis

❓ Q3

Patient found to be pyrexial:

- ▬ A contrast-enhanced MR was performed
- ▬ Selected images—T2W sagittal, T1W sagittal and T1W contrast-enhanced sagittal and T2W axial images—are shown

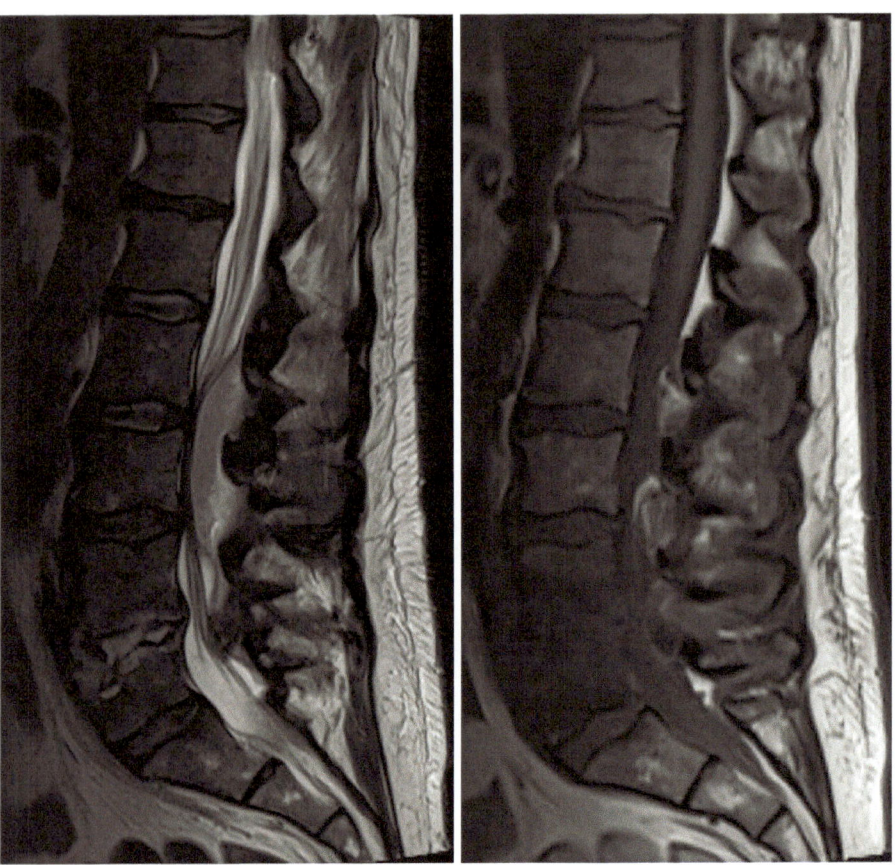

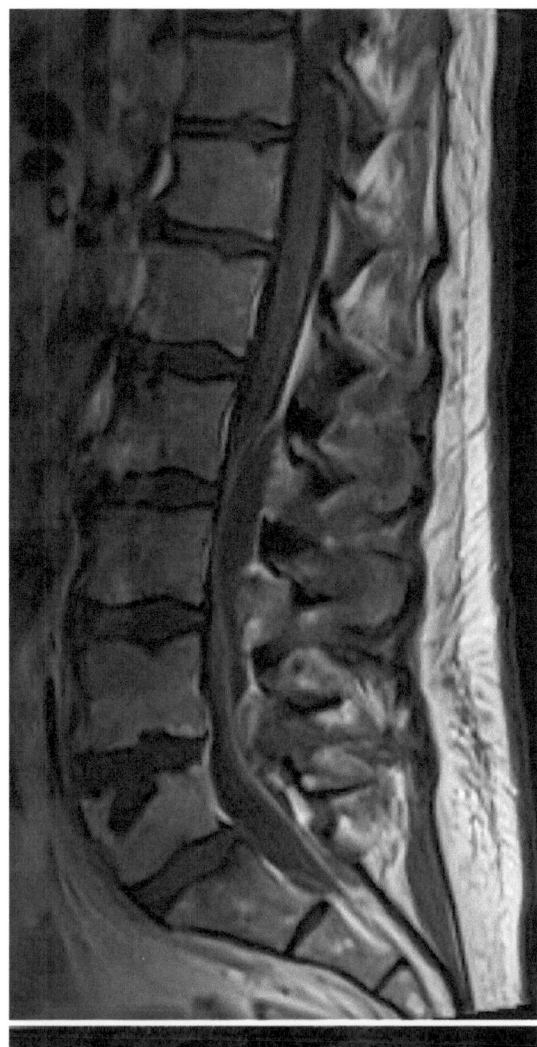

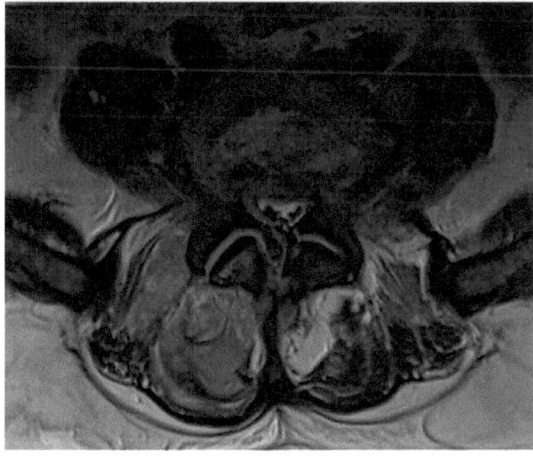

Given the history and imaging findings, what is the most likely diagnosis?
(Multiple answers might be correct.)
1. Modic type III changes
2. Spondylodiscitis
3. Gout
4. Ankylosing spondylitis
5. Diffuse idiopathic skeletal hyperostosis

❓ Q4

Regarding spondylodiscitis, which of the following statements are correct?
(Multiple answers might be correct.)
1. In adults, the infection is thought to start in the disc and extend to involve the endplates
2. Psoas abscesses are seen in pyogenic spondylodiscitis but rarely in tuberculous spondylodiscitis
3. Multilevel involvement spondylodiscitis favours a diagnosis of tuberculous, rather than pyogenic spondylodiscitis
4. Presence of vacuum phenomenon makes a diagnosis of infective spondylodiscitis unlikely
5. Discitis following prostatectomy is thought to be secondary to haematogenous seeding of infection via the artery of Adamkiewicz

CORE

C 1

A 24-year-old football player:
- Swelling of right knee joint after trauma
- He complains about medial compartment of the right knee

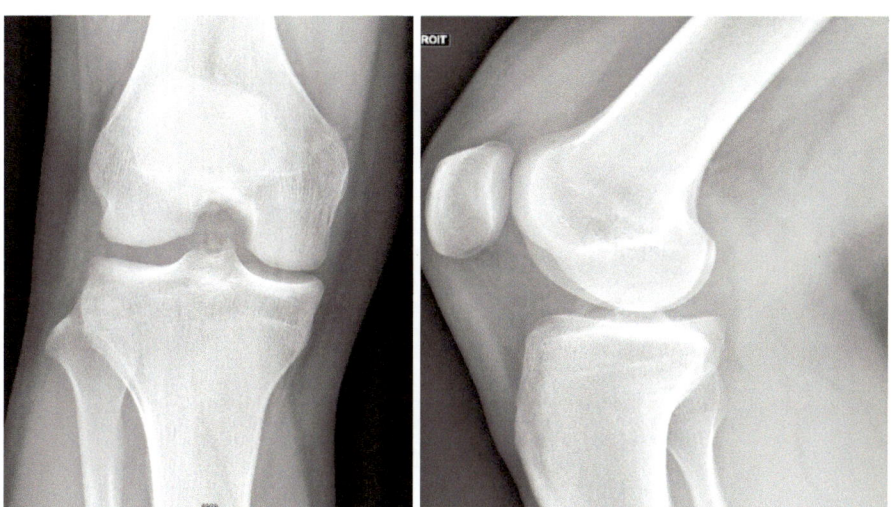

Describe the relevant abnormalities.
Lateral view

_____

_____

_____

Anterior view

_____

_____

_____

List the significant abnormal findings.

_____

_____

_____

8

▪ **Video 8.1**

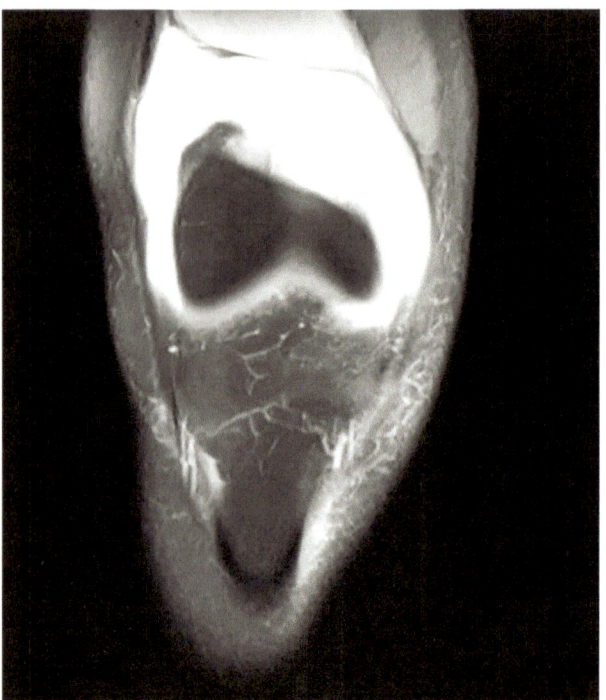

▪ **Video 8.2**

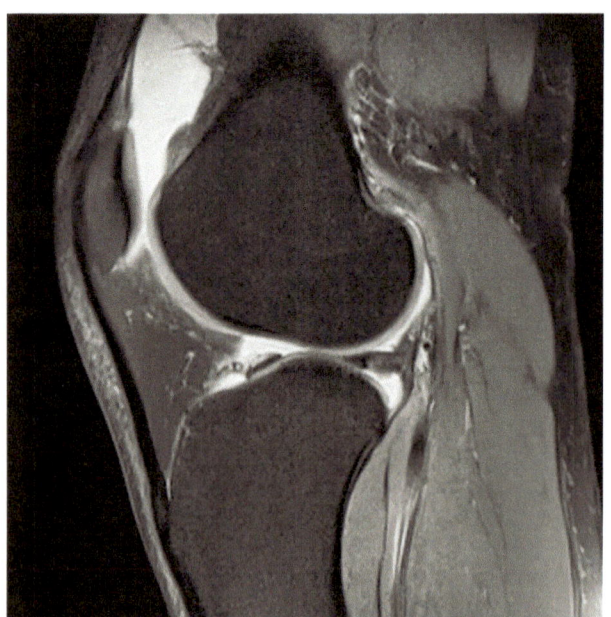

- **Video 8.3**

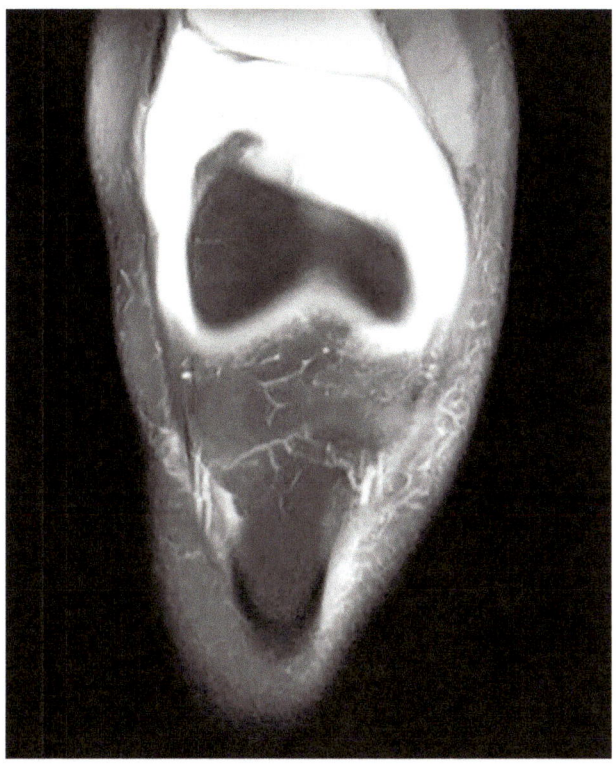

■ **Video 8.4**

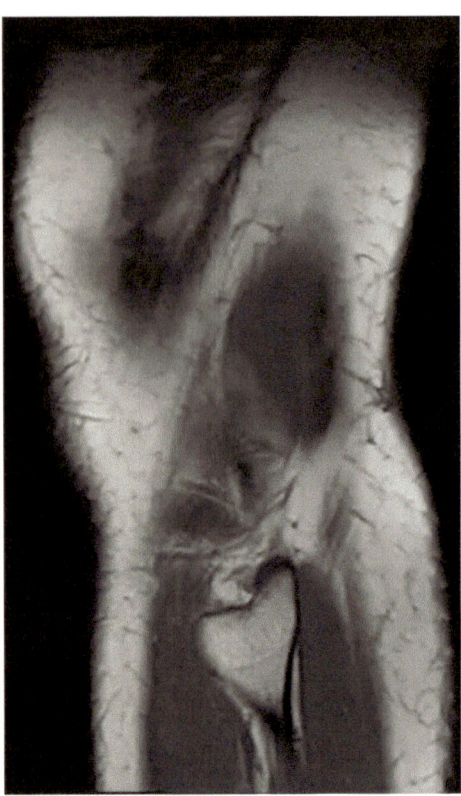

8

❓ Q3
Pick the most correct of the following options to describe the findings:
(Only one option is correct.)
1. Joint effusion, medial meniscal and medial collateral ligament tears
2. Joint effusion, medial meniscal tear and anterior cruciate ligament attachment avulsion
3. Joint effusion, medial meniscal tear and posterior cruciate ligament tear
4. Joint effusion, lateral meniscal tear and posterior cruciate ligament tear
5. Joint effusion, lateral meniscal tear and anterior cruciate ligament attachment avulsion

C 2

A 45-year-old woman:
▬ With pain of the fourth finger of the right hand after a fall

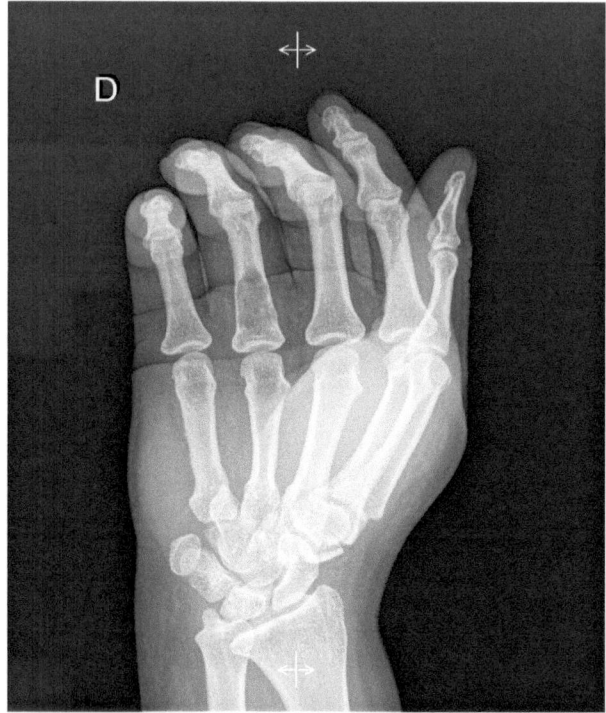

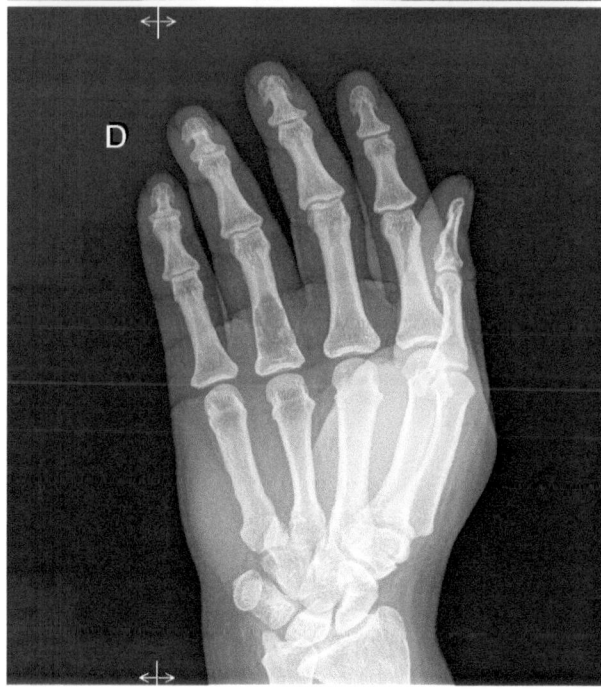

8

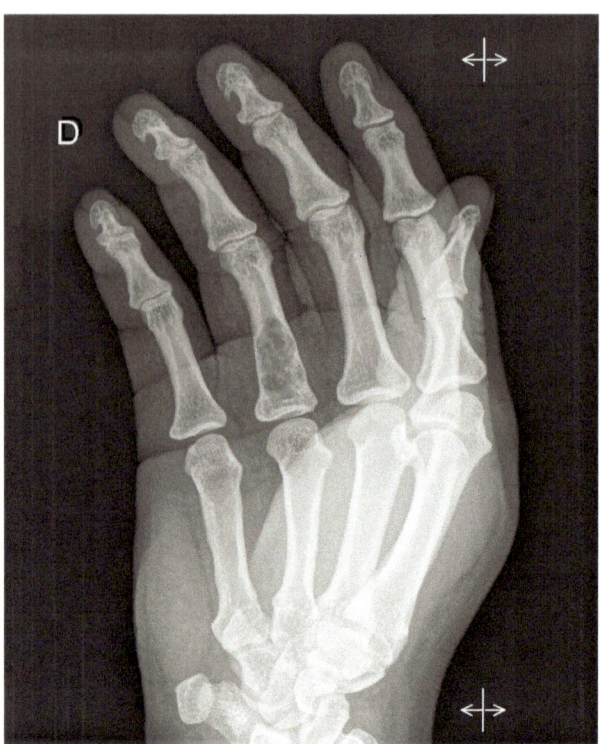

❓ **Q1**
List the significant abnormalities.

_____

_____

_____

❓ **Q2**
One month later, an MRI is performed.

▪ **Video 8.5**

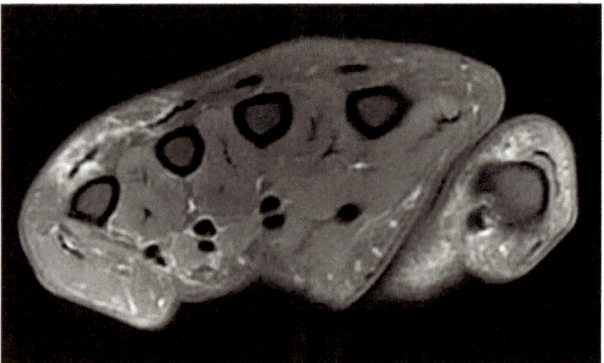

■ **Video 8.6**

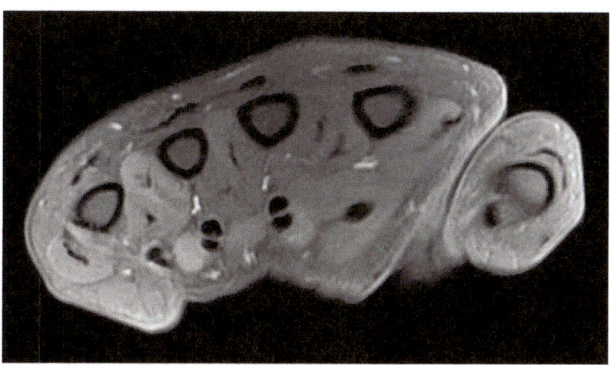

■ **Video 8.7**

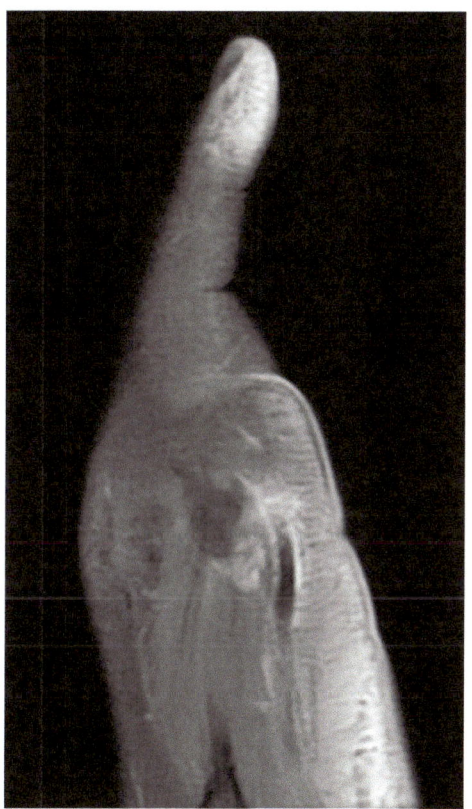

■ **Video 8.8**

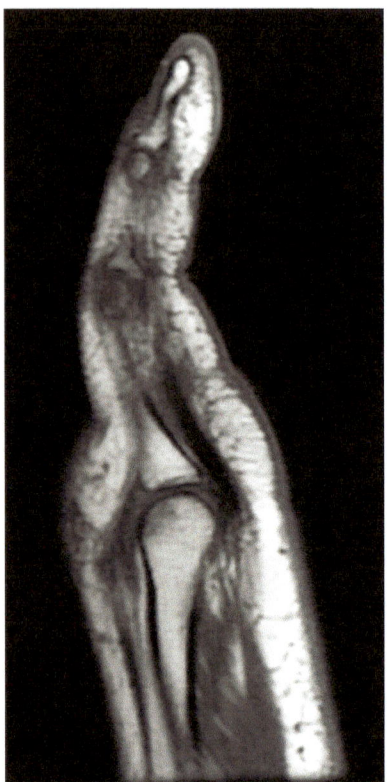

List the most relevant findings.

_____

_____

_____

❓ Q3

What is the most likely diagnosis for this lesion?

(Only one answer is correct.)

1. Solitary enchondroma
2. Chondroblastoma
3. Osteochondroma
4. Fibrous dysplasia
5. Giant cell tumour

Answers

Multiple Response Questions (MRQs)

✅ MRQ 1
1 and 3
Explanation
There is a slight malignant potential of cartilaginous exostoses, about 1%, more frequently (3 to 25%) in case of hereditary multiple exostoses, which is an autosomal dominant disorder, especially for large cartilaginous cap and central location.

✅ MRQ 2
1, 2, 4 and 5
Explanation
All pathologic conditions with joint destruction (rheumatoid arthritis, tuberculosis arthritis) or bone dysplasia (Paget's disease or fibrous dysplasia) can lead to joint deformity, protrusio acetabuli particularly.

✅ MRQ 3
3, 4 and 5
Explanation
The bony element laterally to the cuboid bone is a sesamoid bone usually located within the peroneus longus tendon, thus named peroneum bone. It is rarely symptomatic but can sometimes be fractured in case of direct trauma or can reveal a more distal lesion of the tendon by moving upwards, while the tendon is retracted. Rarely, it is implicated in the genesis of pain and tenosynovitis.

✅ MRQ 4
2 and 5
Explanation
TPD is more frequent in young females with trochlear dysplasia or patella alta. The patella dislocates laterally with impingement of the medial facet with the lateral condyle.

✅ MRQ 5
1, 3 and 4

✅ MRQ 6
1 and 2 and 3
Explanation
Scleroderma involves the hands very frequently causing soft tissue atrophy and fingertips thinning and skin sores. It causes also resorption of ribs and mandibular angle.

✅ MRQ 7
3, 4 and 5
Explanation
Primary hyperparathyroidism usually causes subperiosteal and subchondral bone resorption and chondrocalcinosis. Mixed osteopenia and osteosclerosis and soft tissue calcification are usually seen in secondary hyperparathyroidism with chronic renal insufficiency.

✅ MRQ 8
1 and 2
Explanation
Kienböck's disease (osteonecrosis of the lunate bone) is associated with negative ulnar variance and repetitive loading. It has oedema and sclerotic signal with hypointense T1WI signal and can benefit from conservative treatment, surgical grafting or various lunate excisions depending on the severity of the injury.

✅ MRQ 9
1
Explanation
Osteosarcoma occurs at the metadiaphysis of the long bones, distal femur mainly. The most common form is located intramedullary, and the parosteal form has usually better outcome. This is a lytic lesion with limited amount of calcified matrix, and all kind of periosteal reaction can be seen. However, as it is aggressive, sunburst type or Codman triangle is more frequently found than lamellated reaction.

Short Cases (SCs)

SC 1
✅ Q1
1

✅ Q2
2
Explanation
The lightbulb sign refers to the abnormal AP radiograph appearance of the humeral head in posterior shoulder dislocation. When the humerus dislocates, it also internally rotates such that the head contour projects like a lightbulb when viewed from the front.

Answers

✅ **Q3**
1, 3 and 4

✅ **Q4**
Reverse Bankart /Hill–Sachs lesion

SC 2

✅ **Q1**

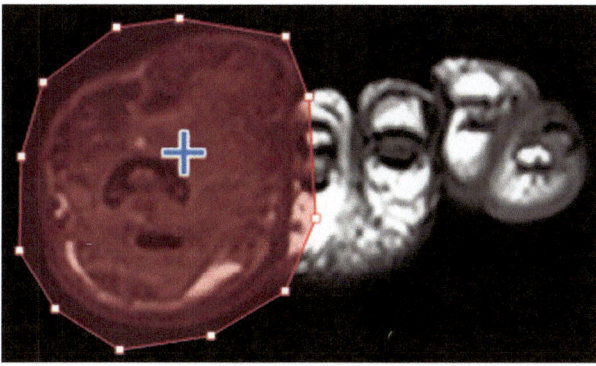

✅ **Q2**
1 and 2

✅ **Q3**
2

✅ **Q4**
1, 3 and 5

SC 3
 Q1

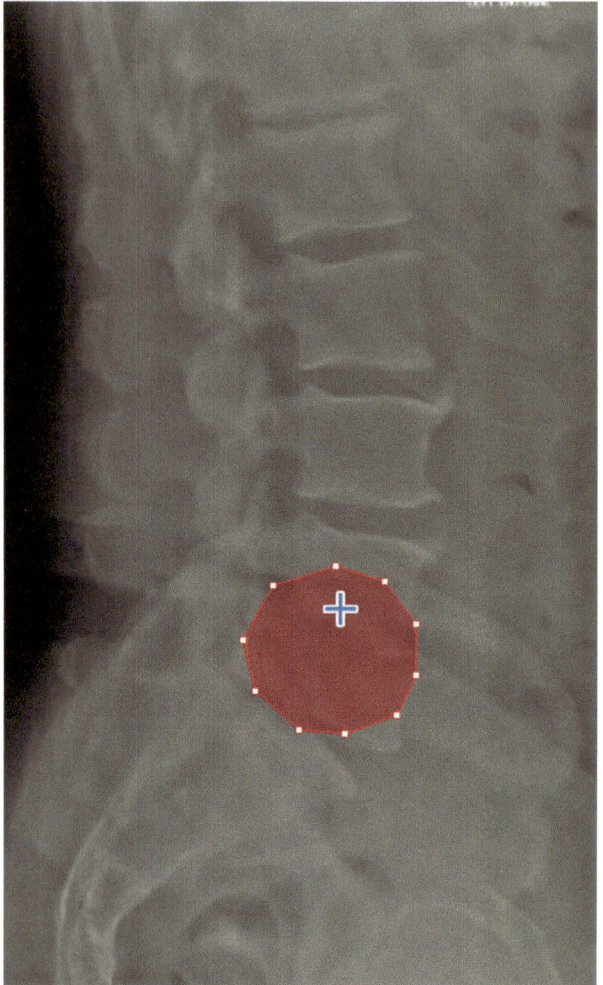

 Q2
2, 3, 4 and 5

 Q3
2

 Q4
3 and 4
Explanation
In adults, haematogenous infection spreads in the edge of the vertebral body endplate and then extends into the disc. On the contrary, disc has blood supply in infants and is the starting point of the infection.

Tuberculous spondylodiscitis often involves multiple adjacent bone levels with frequent soft tissue abscesses.

Vacuum phenomenon in discitis is in favour of degenerative changes.

Discitis following prostatectomy is seeding via Batson's venous plexus.

CORE

C 1

 Q1

Lateral view

Increased density of the suprapatellar recess due to joint effusion

Deep lateral condyle notch (>2 mm)

Abnormal calcified fragment anterior to the spinous process of the tibia (avulsion of the ACL insertion)

Anterior view

Calcified fragment above the tibial eminence, with sharp well-defined margins

 Q2

- Massive joint effusion
- Tear of the medial meniscus and displaced bucket handle fragment along the tibial eminence
- Avulsion of ACL insertion
- Fracture of the tibial spinous process (intercondylar eminence), without bone oedema

 Q3

2

C 2

 Q1

- Well-circumscribed expansile osteolytic lesion in the proximal metaphyseodiaphyseal aspect of the first phalanx of the fourth finger
- Erosion of the endosteal margin of the cortex
- Small foci of calcifications
- Thin linear lucent lines in both sides of cortex indicative of pathological fracture

✅ **Q2**

- Hypointense T1 and hyperintense T2 lesion with heterogeneous pattern
- Mild heterogeneous enhancement predominant in the peripheral aspect of the lesion
- Thin cortical rim
- Minimal residual periosteal reaction due to the fracture callus
- No soft tissue mass

✅ **Q3**

1

Literature

Alyas F, James SL, Davies AM, Saifuddin A. The role of MR imaging in the diagnostic characterisation of appendicular bone tumours and tumour-like conditions. Eur Radiol. 2007;17(10):2675–2686. pub 2007 March 7. Review. PubMed PMID: 17342487.

Aydingöz U, Firat AK, Atay OA, Doral MN. MR imaging of meniscal bucket-handle tears: a review of signs and their relation to arthroscopic classification. Eur Radiol. 2003;13(3):618–625. Epub 2002 September 3. PubMed PMID: 12594567.

De Maeseneer M, Madani H, Lenchik L, et al. Normal anatomy and compression areas of nerves of the foot and ankle: US and MR imaging with anatomic correlation. Radiographics. 2015;35(5):1469–82.

Garcia J, Bianchi S. Diagnostic imaging of tumors of the hand and wrist. Eur Radiol. 2001;11(8):1470–1482. Review. PubMed PMID: 11519560.

Gupta H, Robinson P. Normal shoulder ultrasound: anatomy and technique. Semin Musculoskelet Radiol. 2015;19(3):203–11.

Jaremko JL, Guenther ZD, Jans LB, Macmahon PJ. Spectrum of injuries associated with paediatric ACL tears: an MRI pictorial review. Insights Imaging. 2013;4(3):273–285. Epub 2013 May 9. PubMed PMID: 23657940; PubMed Central PMCID: PMC3675256.

Mellado JM, Ramos A, Salvadó E, Camins A, Calmet J, Saurí A. Avulsion fractures and chronic avulsion injuries of the knee: role of MR imaging. Eur Radiol. 2002;12(10):2463–2473. Epub 2002 Mar 23. Review. PubMed PMID: 12271386.

Mohankumar R, White LM, Naraghi A. Pitfalls and pearls in MRI of the knee. Am J Roentgenol. 2014;203:516–30.

Additional EDiR Preparatory Materials

http://learn.myesr.org

EDiR Preparation Sessions

http://learn.myesr.org
Soft tissue tumours.
Bone tumours.
The bare bones: large joint: the knee.

Neuroradiology

Electronic supplementary material The online version of this chapter
(https://doi.org/10.1007/978-3-030-20066-4_9) contains supplementary material,
which is available to authorized users.

Multiple Response Questions (MRQs)

❓ MRQ 1

Regarding meningiomas, which of the following statements are correct?
(Multiple answers might be correct.)
1. The CSF cleft sign can be seen
2. Meningiomas cannot appear around the optic nerve due to lack of dural sheath
3. Meningiomas typically show ring enhancement
4. 90% of meningiomas occur supratentorially
5. Only 10% of meningiomas show a dural tail sign

❓ MRQ 2

Regarding Chiari type II malformation, which statements are correct?
(Multiple answers might be correct.)
1. Supratentorial abnormalities are uncommon
2. Small posterior fossa
3. It is never associated with hydrocephalus
4. The tectum shows beaking
5. It is nearly always associated with neural tube defect

9

❓ MRQ 3

Regarding multiple sclerosis, which statements are correct?
(Multiple answers might be correct.)
1. Involvement of the U-fibres is necessary to diagnose MS
2. Tumefactive MS typically presents with complete ring enhancement
3. MS-typical regions are periventricular, juxtacortical, infratentorial and spinal cord
4. Multiple sclerosis is a classic example of a primary demyelinating disease
5. Enhancing lesions are indicative of active demyelination and disruption of the blood–brain barrier

❓ MRQ 4

Regarding radiation-induced white matter lesions, which of the following statements are true?
(Multiple answers might be correct.)
1. PET is of no value in distinguishing between tumour recurrence and radiation necrosis
2. Radiation leukoencephalitis typically occurs 6–9 months after treatment
3. Radiation necrosis can be progressive and fatal
4. Radiation necrosis typically presents as an enhancing lesion with mass effect
5. Perfusion MRI helps to differentiate glioblastoma multiforme from radiation necrosis

? MRQ 5

Regarding spinal cord tumours, which of the following statements are correct?
(Multiple answers might be correct.)

1. Spinal cord tumours commonly have cysts and syrinx
2. The most common tumour of the spinal cord is metastasis
3. For evaluation of spinal cord tumours, contrast administration is necessary
4. Spinal cord tumours will typically have spinal cord enlargement
5. Astrocytoma is the most common spinal cord tumour in children

? MRQ 6

9-year-old boy with epilepsy and psychomotor retardation, MRI was performed:

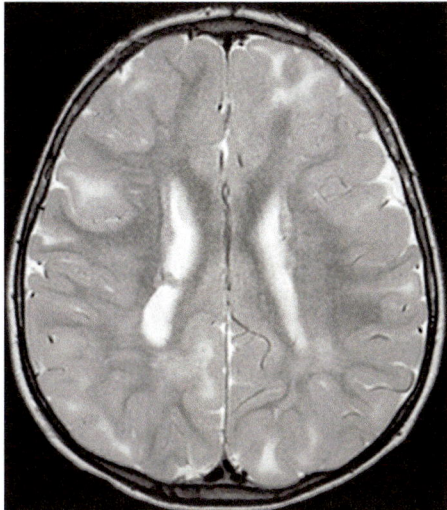 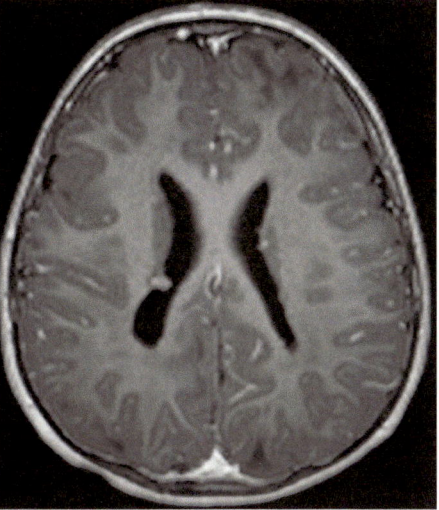

Which statements are correct?
(Multiple answers might be correct.)

1. The foci of high signal intensity in the cortex are metastases
2. Most likely diagnosis is neurofibromatosis type I
3. The subcortical lesions most likely correspond to glioneuronal tubers
4. The periventricular lesions correspond to subependymal glial nodules
5. The subependimal lesions might calcify

❓ MRQ 7
12-year-old female with diabetes insipidus, MRI was performed:

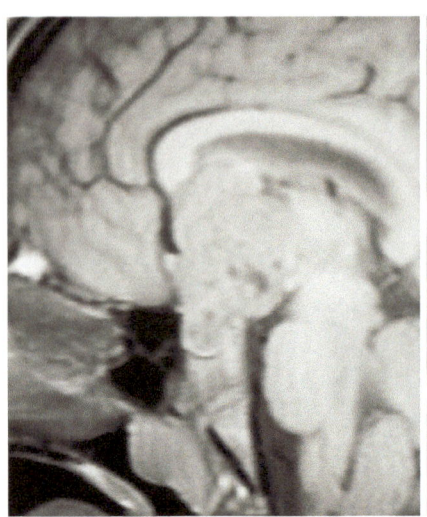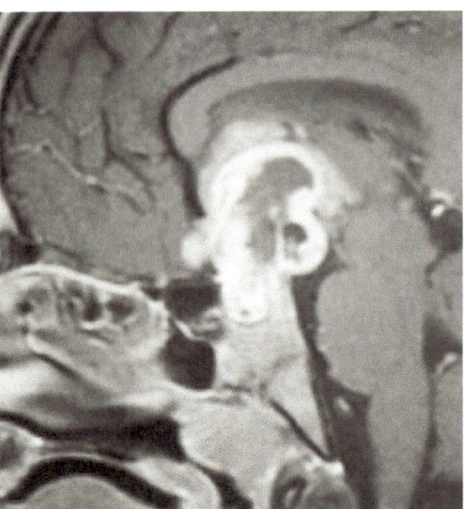

9

Which statements are correct?
(Multiple answers might be correct.)
1. There is a pituitary bright spot
2. The lesion arises from the chiasma
3. The lesion involves the hypothalamus
4. This lesion is aggressive
5. This lesion is most likely a germinoma

❓ MRQ 8
56-year-old female presenting with the worst headache of her life, CT was performed:

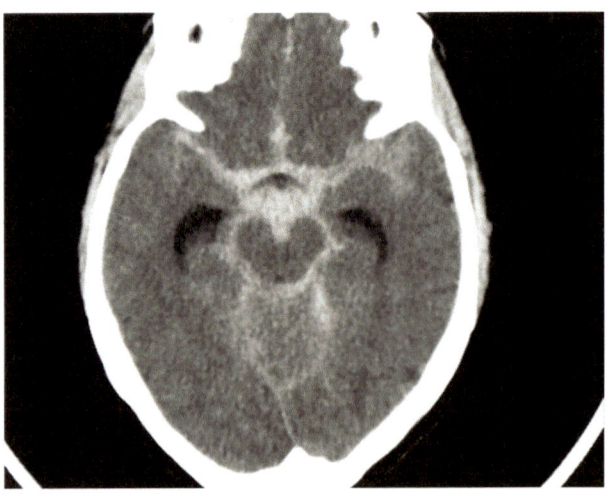

Which of the following are correct?
(Multiple answers might be correct.)
1. There is hydrocephalus
2. There is extensive vascular enhancement
3. Patient is at risk for ischemia
4. Antihypertensive treatment is key in the treatment regimen
5. MRI needs to be performed in the acute phase

❓ **MRQ 9**
Structures that return high signal on T2-weighted MR of the spine include:
(Multiple answers might be correct.)
1. Degenerate disc
2. Arachnoid diverticulum
3. Dorsal root ganglion
4. Tarlov cyst
5. Infected disc (discitis)

Short Cases (SCs)

SC 1

A 64-year-old male:
— With headache and confusion

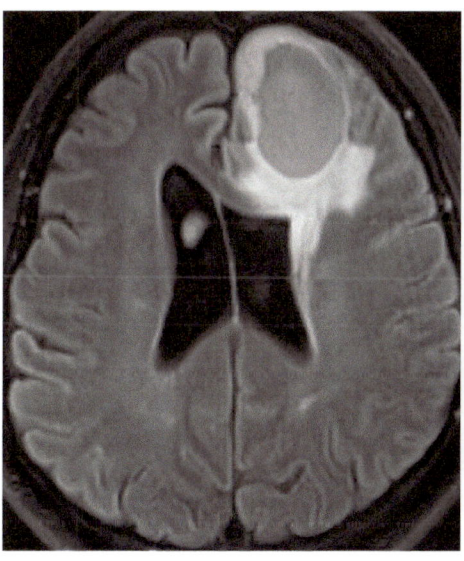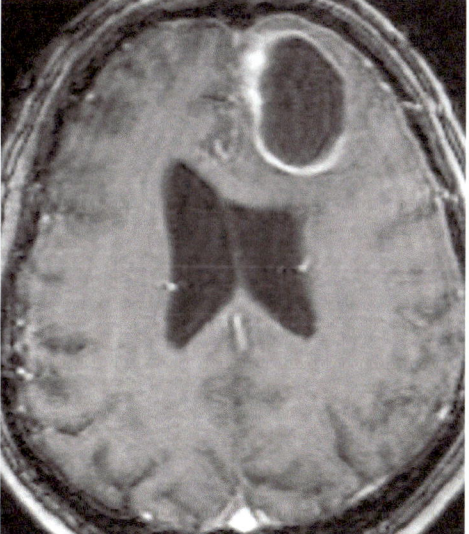

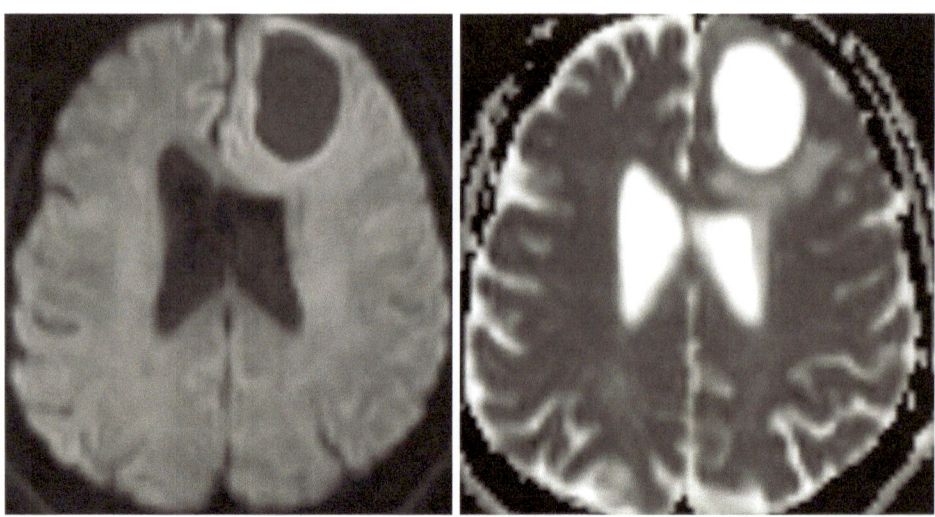

■ ADC

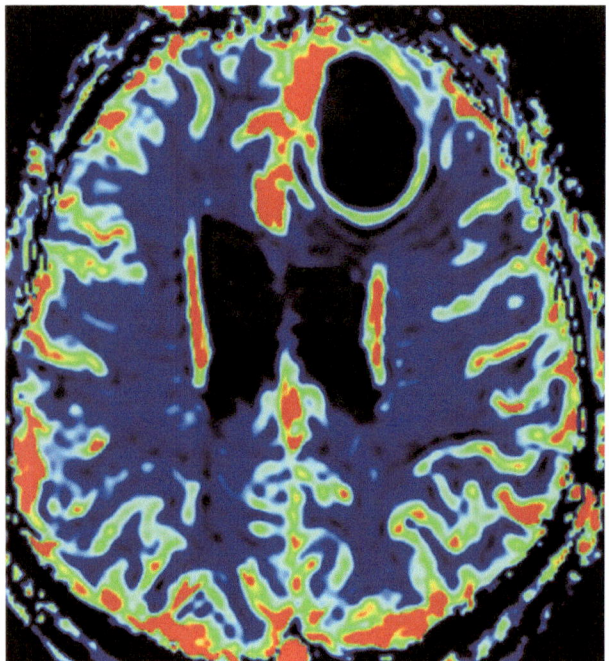

■ CBV

❓ Q1

What is the most likely diagnosis?

(Only one answer is correct.)

1. Cystic metastasis
2. Epidermoid cyst
3. Meningioma
4. Brain abscess
5. Craniopharyngioma

❓ Q2

What course of actions would you take next?

(Multiple answers might be correct.)

1. Whole-body PET-CT
2. Wait and see
3. Biopsy of the lesion
4. Surgical resection
5. Non-enhanced CT to evaluate the osseous structures

SC 2

50-year-old male:

- Spastic legs > arms
- Consanguineous
- Sag T1 is performed

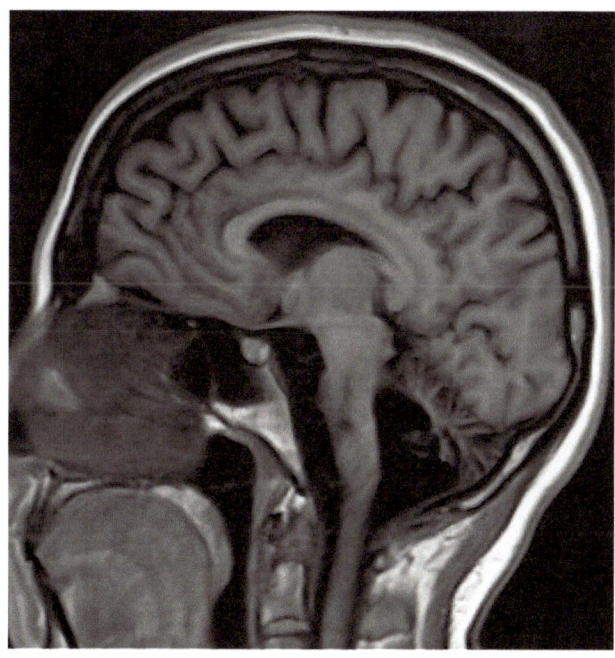

? **Q1**

Indicate the abnormality.

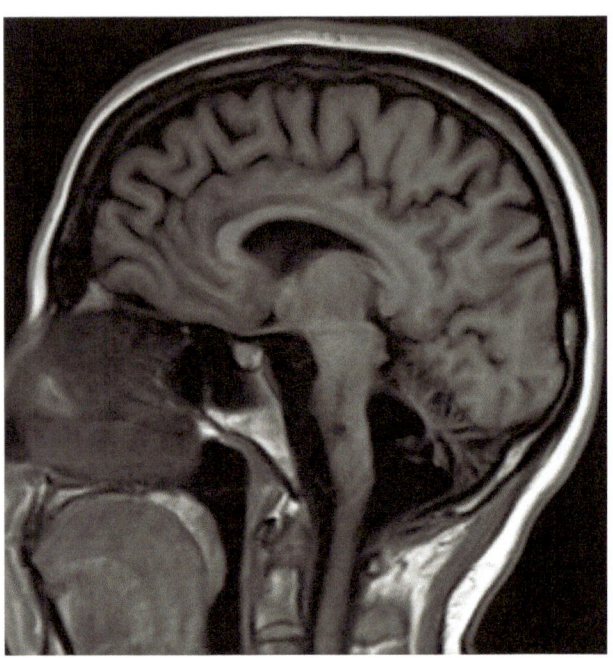

? **Q2**

Differential diagnosis includes:

(Multiple answers might be correct.)

1. Joubert syndrome
2. Multiple system atrophy (MSA)
3. Arachnoid cyst
4. Epidermoid cyst
5. Progressive supranuclear palsy (PSP)

9

❓ Q3
Regarding the images shown:

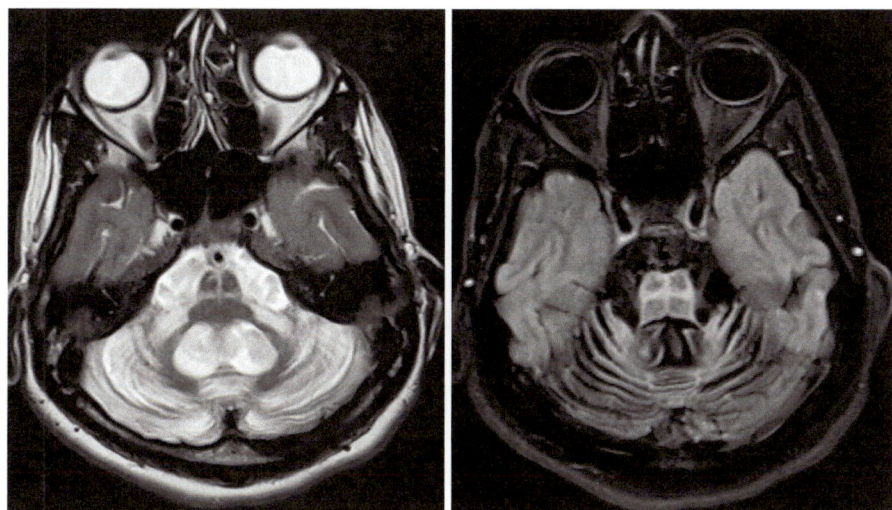

Which of the following statements are correct?
(Multiple answers might be correct.)
1. Most likely diagnosis is MSA
2. There is abnormal signal intensity in the pons
3. Image is at the level of the inferior cerebellar peduncle
4. There is marked cerebellar atrophy
5. There is a lesion in the fourth ventricle

❓ Q4
Concerning the diagnosis, which statements are correct?
(Multiple answers might be correct.)
1. There is atrophy of the middle cerebellar peduncles
2. Treatment involves correction of hyponatremia
3. The brainstem signal abnormality is called "hummingbird sign"
4. Abnormalities in basal ganglia can occur in this disease
5. The cerebellar abnormalities are reversible

SC 3

69-year-old male:
- Fell 6 days ago
- Rhinorrhoea
- CT axial soft tissue and coronal bone window are shown

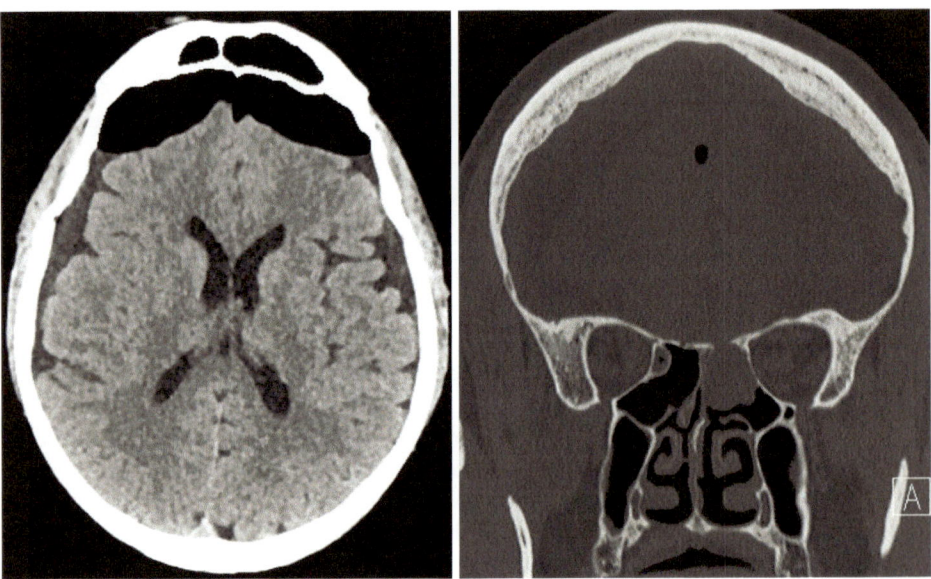

❓ Q1
Indicate the main abnormality.

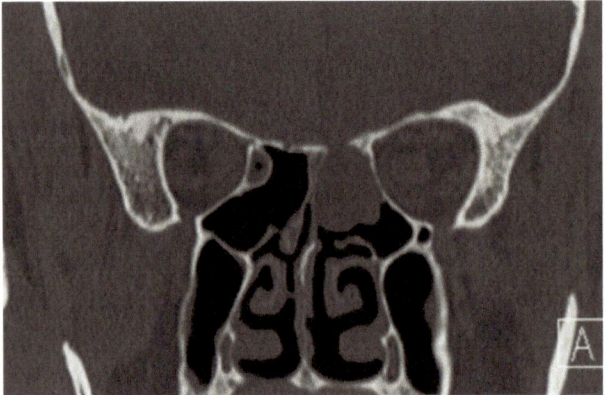

❓ Q2

Differential diagnosis includes:
(Multiple answers might be correct.)
1. Hygroma
2. Air embolus
3. Arachnoid cyst
4. Chronic subdural haematoma
5. Skull base trauma

❓ Q3

CT cisternography was done:

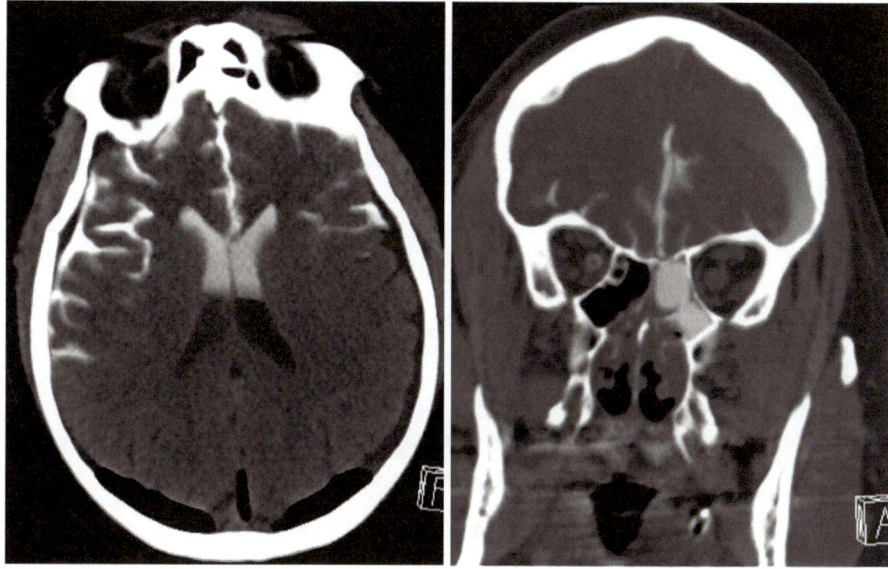

Give the most likely diagnosis.

_____

_____

_____

❓ Q4

Concerning CSF leaks, which of the following statements are correct?
(Multiple answers might be correct.)
1. They can occur after pituitary surgery
2. Patient is at higher risk of meningitis
3. Radionuclide studies can help detect a small leak
4. Pneumocephalus in this case is mainly in the epidural space
5. They can lead to intracranial hypertension

CORE

57-year-old man:
- Reporting "mild" cervical trauma during rugby
- Progressive right hemiparesis since 1 week
- No fever

CT is shown:

- **Video 9.1**

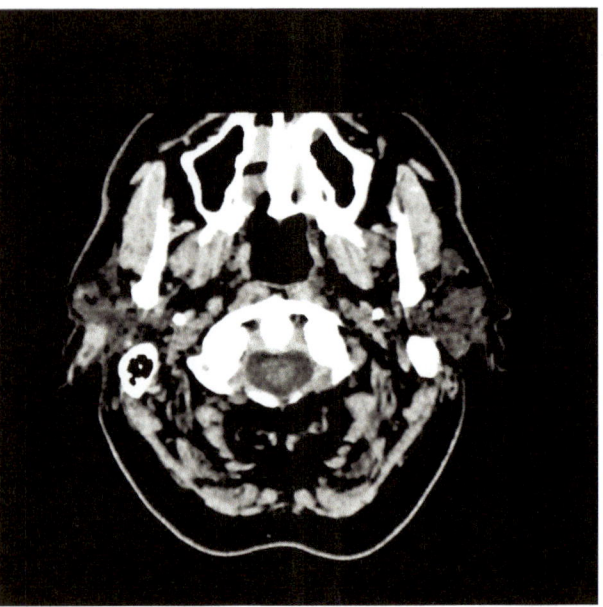

? Q1
Write down TWO relevant cerebral findings.

_____

_____

_____

? Q2

■ **Video 9.2**

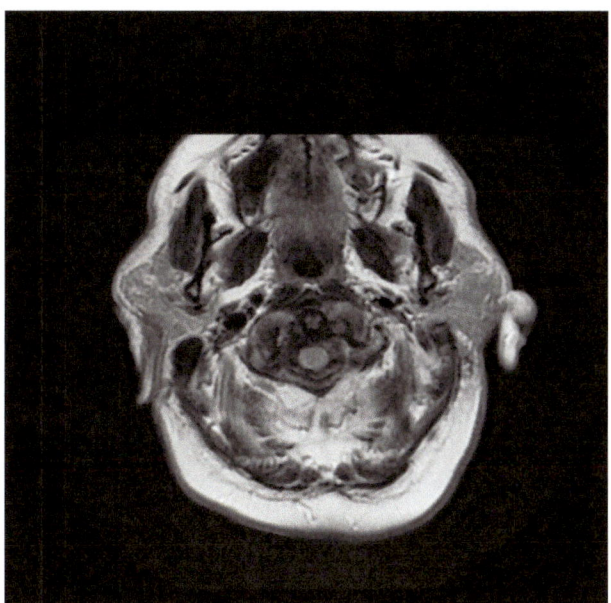

◘ Ax T2 FLAIR

■ **Video 9.3**

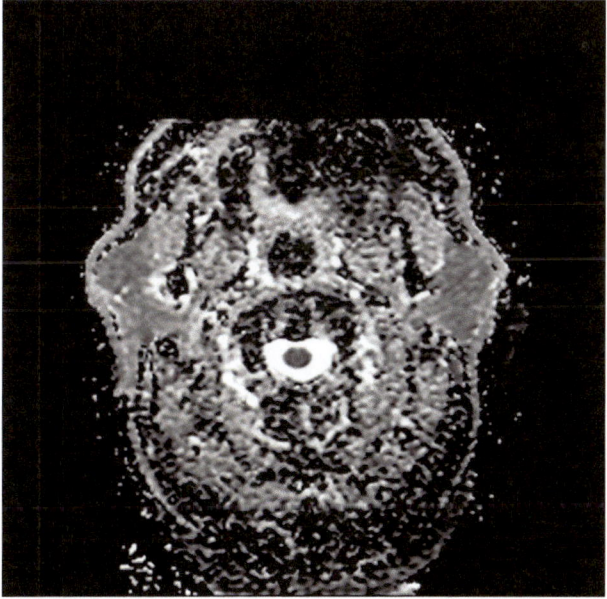

◘ Ax Diffusion

■ **Video 9.4**

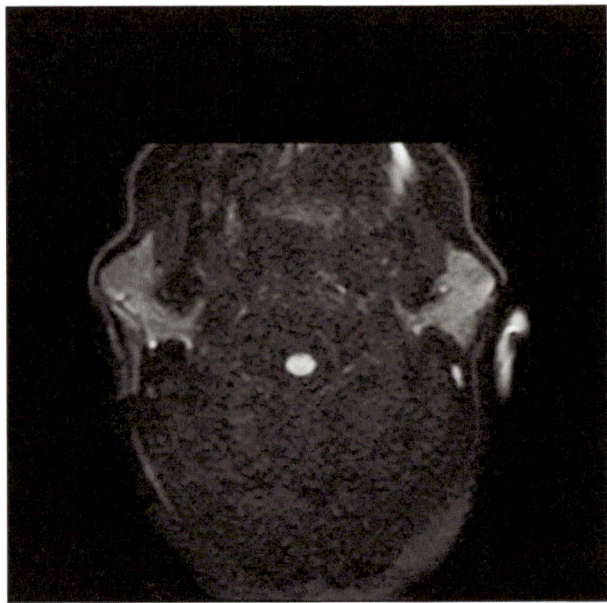

9

◼ Ax ADC

■ **Video 9.5**

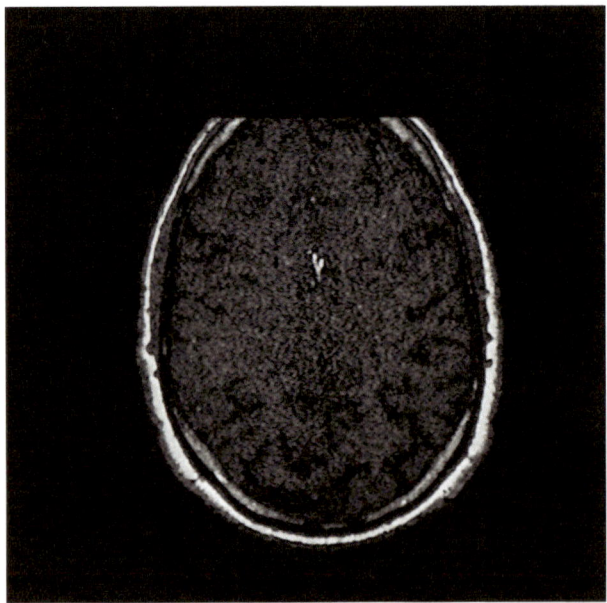

◼ Ax TOF

■ **Video 9.6**

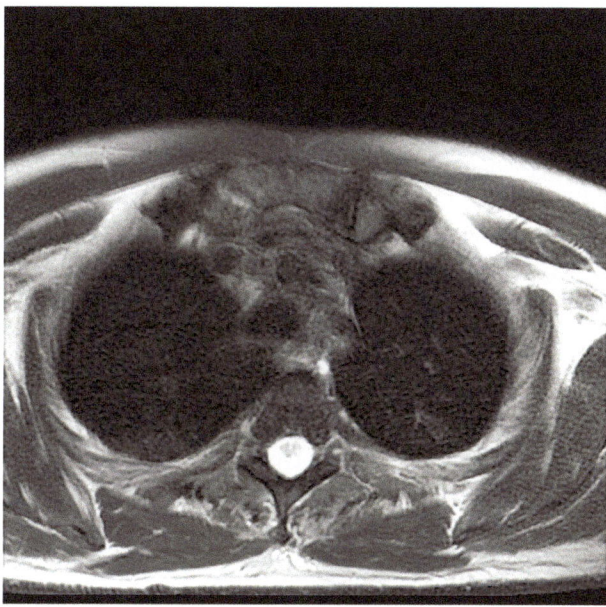

◘ **Ax T2 FS**

Describe the findings.

_____

_____

_____

❓ **Q3**
Which is the most likely diagnosis?

_____

_____

_____

Answers

Multiple Response Questions (MRQs)

 MRQ 1

1 and 4

Explanation

Meningiomas are extra-axial tumours, arising from the dura. Between the meningioma and the underlying brain parenchyma, often a rim of CSF can be seen, called "the CSF cleft sign", which is considered a sign of extra-axial location [1]. Other signs of extra-axial location are the fact that parenchymal grey matter is abutting the meningioma and the brain parenchyma is compressed like an "accordion". The vast majority of meningiomas occur supratentorially, primarily around the convexity or on the falx. The dural tail sign occurs as a result of thickening and enhancement of the dura and is most often seen adjacent to a meningioma [2]. A dural tail sign is seen in > 50% of meningiomas. Meningiomas typically show solid intense enhancement on both CT and MRI [3]. The optic nerve contains a dural sheath which can develop meningiomas. These typically present with parallel thickening and enhancement around the optic nerve, called the "tram track" sign [4].

9

MRQ 2

2, 4 and 5

Explanation

A Chiari type II malformation is a congenital malformation of the hindbrain associated with a neural tube closure defect, usually a lumbar myelomeningocele. The typical radiological features are a small posterior fossa with a descent of the brainstem and cerebellar tonsils through the foramen magnum, in combination with the spinal dysraphism. It is associated with a large number of other abnormalities, including dysgenesis of the corpus callosum, hydrocephalus and tectal beaking. The latter is an abnormal morphology of the midbrain due to fusion of the colliculi into a single beak pointing posteriorly.

As a differential diagnosis, the Chiari type I malformation is not associated with a myelomeningocele, and a Chiari type III malformation shows an encephalocele.

MRQ 3

3, 4 and 5

Explanation

Demyelinating disorders of the central nervous system are characterised by the breakdown of myelin, with or without preservation of the associated axons. Primary demyelinating diseases typically involve loss of myelin with relative sparing of axons. Multiple sclerosis is the most common primary demyelinating disorder. Secondary demyelinating disorders are characterised by damage to neurons or axons with consequent also breakdown of myelin. Secondary demyelinating diseases are associated with a wide variety of conditions, including infections, nutritional deficiencies, toxicity, genetic abnormalities and vascular insult. Wallerian degeneration is a well-known example of secondary demyelination.

The 2017 McDonald diagnostic criteria for multiple sclerosis are clinical, radiographic and laboratory criteria used in the diagnosis of multiple sclerosis.

Tumefactive MS is a variant of multiple sclerosis, presenting as a large brain lesion with usually less mass effect than would be expected for its size. After gadolinium injection, there can be some peripheral enhancement, often with an incomplete ring ("horseshoe" or open ring enhancement). This type of enhancement can distinguish tumefactive MS from brain gliomas or abscesses.

✅ MRQ 4

2, 3, 4 and 5

Explanation

Distinguishing residual/recurrent neoplasm from radiation-induced necrosis is difficult using conventional MRI alone, as necrosis shows enhancement patterns which may mimic (high-grade) tumour. Perfusion MRI, PET or SPECT may help distinguish recurrent tumour from radiation-induced necrosis, as radiation necrosis generally shows lower perfusion (lower cerebral blood volume) and lower FDG uptake than tumour recurrence. Symptoms associated with radionecrosis are non-specific and can mimic tumour recurrence (seizures, intracranial hypertension and focal neurological deficit). Radiation necrosis can be progressive and fatal.

Acute toxicity from brain irradiation occurs within days or at most first few weeks of therapy (i.e. brain oedema). Early delayed toxicity occurs within weeks to 3 months of treatment. Pseudoprogression can be detected during this subacute phase or later (even within 6–9 months), and it is due to a florid treatment effect with oedema and enhancing lesions.

Late toxicity (i.e. leukoencephalitis, vasculopathy, brain tumours) occurs any time after 90 days from brain irradiation (usually 6–9 months or, sometimes, decades later).

✅ MRQ 5

1, 3, 4 and 5

Explanation

Intramedullary neoplasms have three general characteristics on MRI: they cause spinal cord expansion; they have high signal on T2-weighted images, and most of them show at least some contrast enhancement.

The vast majority (95%) of intramedullary tumours are glial tumours. Astrocytomas are the most common in children, whereas ependymomas are the most common intramedullary neoplasm in adults. Intramedullary metastases are rare.

Approximately 70% of intramedullary tumours are associated with cysts which can be tumoural or non-tumoural. Syringomyelia occurs in approximately 50% of all intramedullary tumours but is most frequently associated with haemangioblastomas.

9

✅ MRQ 6

3, 4 and 5

Explanation

Tuberous sclerosis, also known as Bourneville–Pringle syndrome, is an inherited tumour disorder from the group of neurocutaneous disorders (or phacomatoses) which shows the development of multiple hamartomas in many organ systems. The classic clinical triad, only seen in approximately 30% of cases, consists of facial angiofibromas, mental retardation and seizures. Since this triad is only seen in a minority of patients, several other diagnostic criteria are defined, including several features outside the central nervous system.

Abnormalities in the brain that typically can be seen are as follows:
- Cortical/subcortical tubers:
  - Can be hyperintense in T1WI
  - Frequently calcify
- Subependymal hamartomas:
  - Majority show calcification after early childhood.
  - Enhancement is possible and is not a reliable feature for distinction from SEGA.
- White matter abnormalities:
  - Cystic lesions
  - Radial bands from periventricular white matter to the subcortical region
- Subependymal giant cell astrocytoma (SEGA or SGCA):
  - Enhancing mass, usually near the foramen of Monro
  - Can induce obstructive hydrocephalus
  - Shows slow growth, a distinguishing feature from subependymal hamartomas

✅ MRQ 7

3, 4 and 5

Explanation

MRI demonstrates a lobulated mass centred in the suprasellar region with large internal cystic areas and vivid contrast enhancement of the solid component. It is an aggressive lesion, which invades adjacent structures like hypothalamus, third ventricle, pituitary sella and frontal lobe. Optic chiasm cannot be recognised. It extends towards the interpeduncular cistern and has no cleavage plane with the midbrain. Pituitary gland is totally invaded so the bright spot that represents the posterior pituitary (neurohypophysis) is not visible.

This lesion in a 12-year-old woman is most likely a germinoma as they are tumours that mainly occur in children and young adults. Approximately 80–90% of patients with central nervous system germ cell are less than 25 years old, with the incidence peaking at 10–14 years. They generally occur in midline locations, with 80% or more arising in structures around the third ventricle. Most commonly, they arise in the region of the pineal gland, followed by the suprasellar region. Tandem lesions affecting both the suprasellar and pineal regions have also been reported in 16–21% of cases. Suprasellar germinomas often have ill-defined margins and irregular shape. They commonly show necrosis, cysts and haemorrhage inside the tumour (nearly 40%), but rarely calcification. On MRI it appears as a solid mass that is isointense or hyperintense relative to grey matter, with prominent enhancement or heterogeneous enhancement if cysts are present.

✅ MRQ 8

1 and 3

Explanation

This non-contrast CT image shows hyperdense material, compatible with blood, in the subarachnoid space (suprasellar cistern, basal cisterns, Sylvian fissure, prepontine cistern). In 85% of spontaneous subarachnoid haemorrhages, rupture of a berry aneurysm of intracranial arteries is the cause. CT angiography is therefore indicated in the acute phase. A common complication is hydrocephalus, shown in this image as widening of the temporal horns. Patients are also at risk for cerebral vasospasm causing delayed cerebral ischaemia. This is prevented using triple H therapy (**H**aemodilution, **H**ypertension, **H**ypervolemia).

✅ MRQ 9

2, 4 and 5

Explanation

Generally, degenerative changes of the disc affect hydration and elasticity of the cartilaginous endplate, annulus fibrosis and nucleus pulposus, with signal intensity on T2 reflecting lower water content (lower T2 signal intensity).

Spinal arachnoid diverticula are formed by the partial seclusion of the subarachnoid space and contain CSF and hence have high internal signal intensity on T2-weighted imaging. These diverticula occurred more frequently in the dorsal than the cervical spinal canal. Large ones may produce symptoms by gravitational traction upon the spinal cord.

The dorsal root ganglion is an enlargement of the dorsal root of spinal nerves representing the cell bodies of the primary somatosensory neurons. Signal intensity on T2-weighted images is similar to the rest of the nerve root, i.e. relatively low. The dorsal root ganglia may enhance after the administration of gadolinium. This enhancement must not be confused with a tumoural process (e.g. schwannoma).

Tarlov cysts, also called perineural cysts, are CSF-filled dilatations of the nerve root sheath at the dorsal root ganglion (posterior nerve root sheath). They show high signal intensity on T2.

An infected disc (discitis) is characterised on imaging by high signal intensity on T2-weighted imaging (due to oedema) and enhancement on T1+Gd. If apart from the disc also associated vertebrae are affected by infection, this is called spondylodiscitis.

Short Cases (SCs)

SC 1

 Q1

1

 Q2

1, 3 and 4

Explanation

Left frontal cystic lesion with peripheral enhancing rim, more marked on the medial border and surrounding oedema compressing the adjacent lateral ventricle and effacing sulci.

The lesion is an intra-axial mass, so it cannot be a meningioma (located extra-axially) or an epidermoid cyst (intracisternal mass) or a craniopharyngioma (sellar-suprasellar mass).

There is no evidence of restriction of diffusion, typical of brain abscess or of epidermoid cyst.

The sparing of the cortex, the surrounding white matter oedema and the relatively low CBV are some subtle features that can help differentiating metastasis from necrotic GBM.

The next actions that could be taken are as follows:

- Spectroscopy MR for DD with GBM. In metastasis, there is no elevation of choline peak within the peritumoural oedema
- Body PET-CT, which may show systemic lesions/primary tumour in case of a cerebral metastasis
- Biopsy of the lesion for defining the final therapeutic planning

Wait and see cannot be an option since the survival can be less than 1 month without treatment, and it is strictly related to the diagnosis. Surgical resection is not indicated in all cases, and non-enhanced computed tomography (NECT) has a limited additional diagnostic value (only for osteolytic skull lesions, well detected also by PET-CT).

9

SC 2

✅ **Q1**

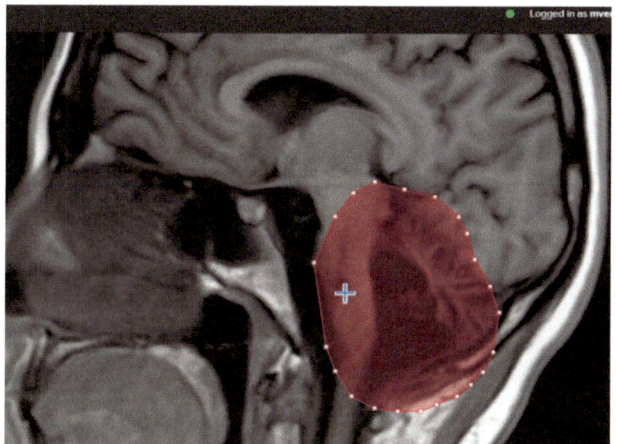

✅ **Q2**

1 and 2

✅ **Q3**

1, 2 and 4

✅ **Q4**

1 and 4

Explanation

The images show a marked atrophy of the cerebellum (including the vermis) and brainstem (more specifically the pons), with also marked atrophy of cerebellar peduncles. The pons shows a typical cross-like sign on T2w images, called "hot cross bun sign".

Multiple system atrophy (MSA) is a sporadic progressive neurodegenerative disorder which usually presents in the fifth or sixth decade with either predominant cerebellar symptoms (MSA-C) or predominant parkinsonian symptoms (MSA-P). Typical radiological findings:

MSA-C:

- Atrophy of the pons, cerebellum, olivary nuclei an middle cerebellar peduncles
- Hot cross bun sign: hyperintense signal on T2WI in a cruciform shape in the pons due to degeneration of the transverse pontocerebellar fibres (not specific for MSA)

MSA-P:

- Reduced volume of the putamen
- Abnormal high signal intensity on T2WI in a rim surrounding the putamen

SC 3
✓ Q1

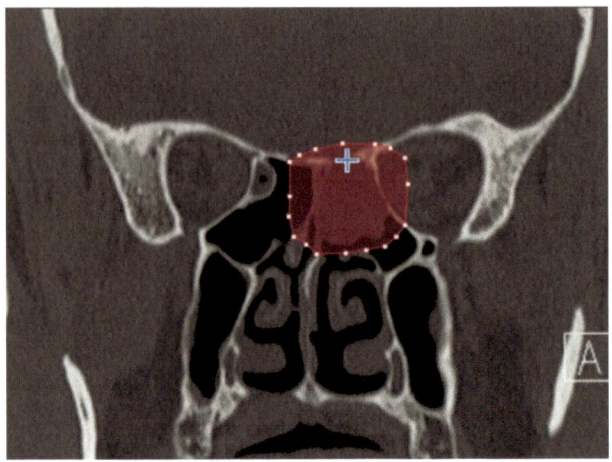

✓ Q2
5

✓ Q3
Skull base fracture with CSF leak

✓ Q4
1, 2 and 3

Explanation

Large osseous defect in the cribriform plate after base skull trauma that can be visualised on coronal bone window CT. Secondary there is a tension pneumocephalus in subdural space causing mass effect over the underlying brain parenchyma.

CSF leak occurs when there is both an osseous defect and a tear of the closely adherent dura, leading to spill of CSF from the subarachnoid space into the sinonasal cavity.

Trauma is the most common cause, but CSF leaks can arise from a number of causes, including congenital malformation, connective tissue disorders, malignant nasopharyngeal and skull base tumours and as a complication of cranial base surgical procedures, e.g. pituitary surgeries, septoplasty or endoscopic surgery.

Communication of the CSF space with the bacterial flora of the nasal or middle ear cavities can result in meningitis, reportedly in up to 50% of cases, if the leak is not repaired. Another common complication is intracranial hypotension, a condition that often presents as a positional headache.

CT cisternography (CTc) is currently the gold standard for diagnosing CSF leaks. It is performed after injecting contrast intrathecally. CSF rhinorrhoea is demonstrated as contrast leakage through the nasal cavity. CTc has a sensitivity of 80% for active CSF leaks, but when no active leak is present, CTc is inferior to high-resolution CT. Radionuclide studies have higher sensitivity in diagnosing leaks but have poor anatomic resolution.

CORE

 Q1
1. SAH (subarachnoid haemorrhage) on the left: ambient cistern, temporal and parasagittal
2. Left FRONTAL paraventricular hypodensities

 Q2
1. T2-Flair: subarachnoid space hyperintensities (left)
2. TOF: left carotid and left middle cerebral arteries non-visible
3. DWI: several ischaemic subacute (no ADC restriction) foci within the anterior watershed area
4. T2 FS: haematoma within the wall of the internal carotid artery (note: most people will do t1 fatsat for dissection, not t2 fatsat)

 Q3
Posttraumatic cervical carotid artery dissection, subacute intracranial ischaemic lesions of the watershed areas and several regions of SAH on the left hemisphere

Literature

Bonatti M, Vezzali N, Ferro F, Manfredi R, Oberhofer N, Bonatti G. Blunt cerebrovascular injury: diagnosis at whole-body MDCT for multi-trauma. Insights Imaging. 2013;4(3):347–55.

Campero A, Ajler P, Emmerich J, Goldschmidt E, Martins C, Rhoton A. Brain sulci and gyri: a practical anatomical review. J Clin Neurosci. 2014;21:2219–25. Epub 2014 August 3.

Dekeyzer S, De Kock I, Nikoubashman O, et al. "Unforgettable" – a pictorial essay on anatomy and pathology of the hippocampus. Insights Imaging. 2017;8(2):199–212.

Filippi M, Rocca MA, Ciccarelli O, et al. MRI criteria for the diagnosis of multiple sclerosis: MAGNIMS consensus guidelines. Lancet Neurol. 2016;15(3):292–303.

Gomez CK, Schiffman SR, Bhatt AA. Radiological review of skull lesions. Insights Imaging. 2018;9(5):857–82.

Muto M, Frauenfelder G, Senese R, Zeccolini F, Schena E, Giurazza F, Jäger HR. Dynamic susceptibility contrast (DSC) perfusion MRI in differential diagnosis between radionecrosis and neoangiogenesis in cerebral metastases using rCBV, rCBF and K2. Radiol Med. 2018;123(7):545 52.

Ryan M, Ibrahim M, Parmar HA. Secondary demyelination disorders and destruction of white matter. Radiol Clin North Am. 2014;52(2):337–54. Epub 2013 December 15.

Soussain C, Ricard D, Fike JR, Mazeron JJ, Psimaras D, Delattre JY. CNS complications of radiotherapy and chemotherapy. Lancet. 2009;374(9701):1639–51.

Additional EDiR Preparatory Materials

http://learn.myesr.org

EDiR Preparatory Sessions

http://learn.myesr.org
Imaging in brain tumours.
Cortical anatomy and primary functional areas.
Pattern recognition in neuroradiology.

Paediatric Radiology

© European Board of Radiology (EBR) 2019
J. Babar et al., *EDiR - The Essential Guide*, https://doi.org/10.1007/978-3-030-20066-4_10

Multiple Response Questions (MRQs)

? **MRQ 1**
A 13-year-old boy, chronic back pain with kyphosis:

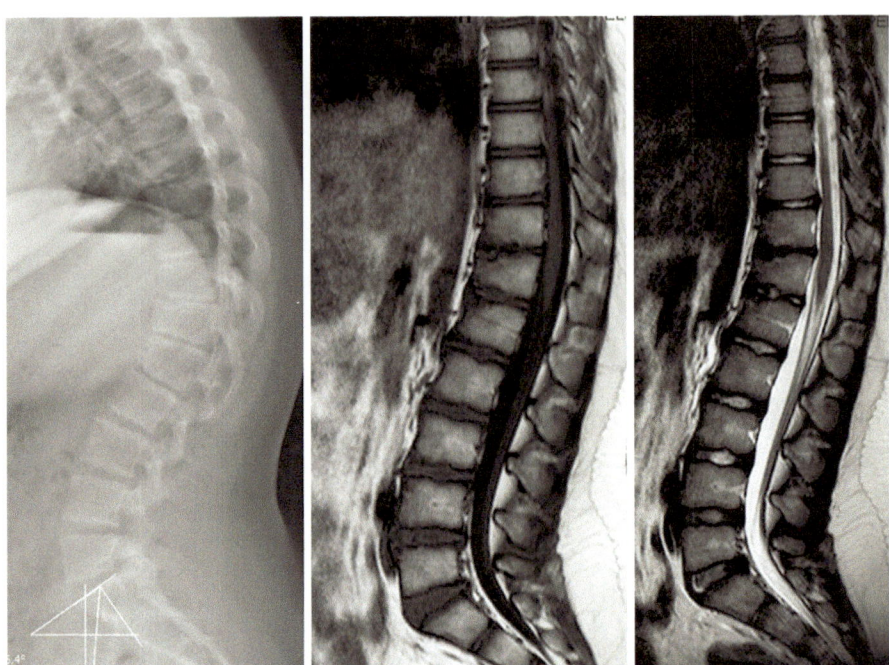

Which of the following statements are correct regarding these images?
(Multiple answers might be correct.)
1. There is narrowing of intervertebral disc spaces of the kyphotic segment
2. Vertebral endplate irregularities are due to extensive disc invagination
3. Kyphosis is in relation to osteoporosis
4. The most likely diagnosis is Scheuermann's disease
5. Kyphosis is related to the wedge-shaped vertebra

10

❓ MRQ 2

Neonate with respiratory distress at birth. After resuscitation, umbilical catheter was inserted, and X-ray was performed soon after:

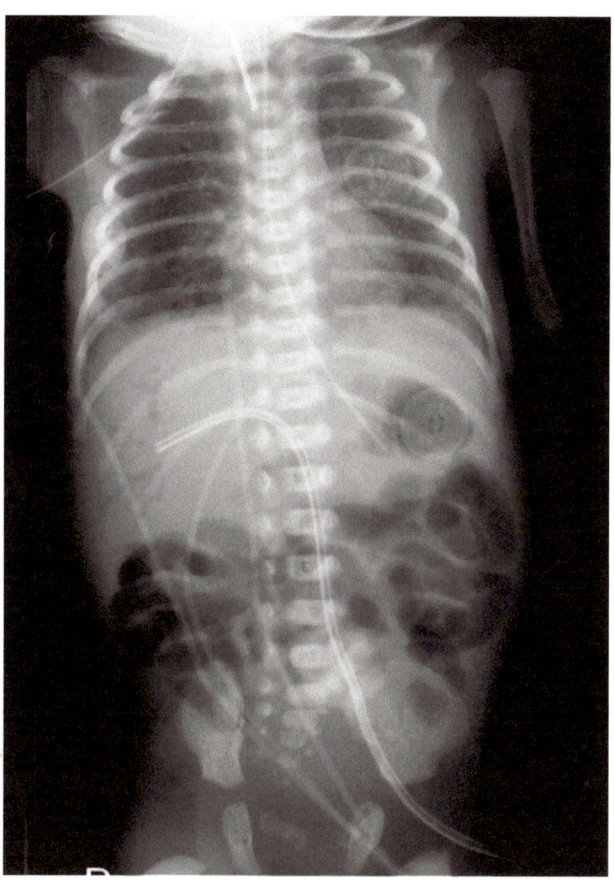

Which of the following statements are correct?
(Multiple answers might be correct.)
1. The umbilical catheter is a venous one
2. Gas within the liver area is consistent with pneumobilia
3. Necrotising enterocolitis is the most likely diagnosis
4. The tracheal tube is well positioned
5. The umbilical catheter is well positioned

❓ MRQ 3

Regarding abdominal cystic lesions in neonates, which of the following sentences are correct?

(Multiple answers might be correct.)

1. Ovarian cysts are the most common cystic lesion found in neonate girls
2. Intestinal duplication cysts have multilayered wall
3. Large multiloculated cysts of undetermined origin are most likely vascular lymphatic malformations
4. The origin of large cysts can be easily established by ultrasound
5. Simple renal cysts represent a very frequent finding

❓ MRQ 4

In a complete duplex urinary collecting system, which of the following statements are correct?

(Multiple answers might be correct.)

1. The pelviureteric junction obstruction is more frequent in the lower moiety
2. The kidney with duplex urinary collecting system is larger than the kidney with a single collecting system
3. The ureterocele is more frequently associated with the lower moiety ureter
4. Vesicoureteral reflux has a higher incidence in the upper moiety than in the lower moiety
5. The ureter of the upper pelvicalyceal system has a more caudal and medial implantation than the normal position

10

❓ MRQ 5

Recognised causes of a calvarial mass in children include:

(Multiple answers might be correct.)

1. Fibrous dysplasia
2. Epidermoid cyst
3. Chronic subdural haematoma
4. Langerhans cell histiocytosis
5. Haemangioma

Short Cases (SCs)

SC 1

An 18-month-old boy:
- With limping for 1 week
- One episode with fever 10 days ago
- No articular swelling is observed

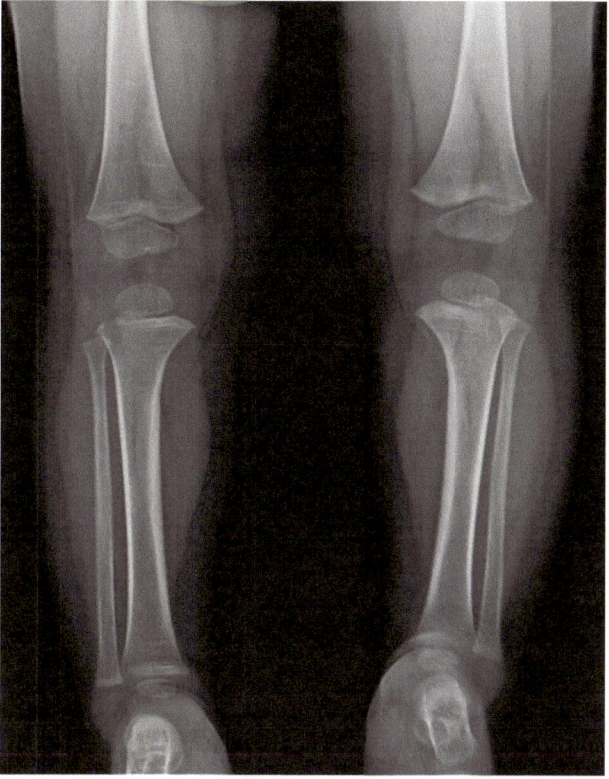

▫ AP view of the lower limbs

❓ Q1

Indicate the abnormality.

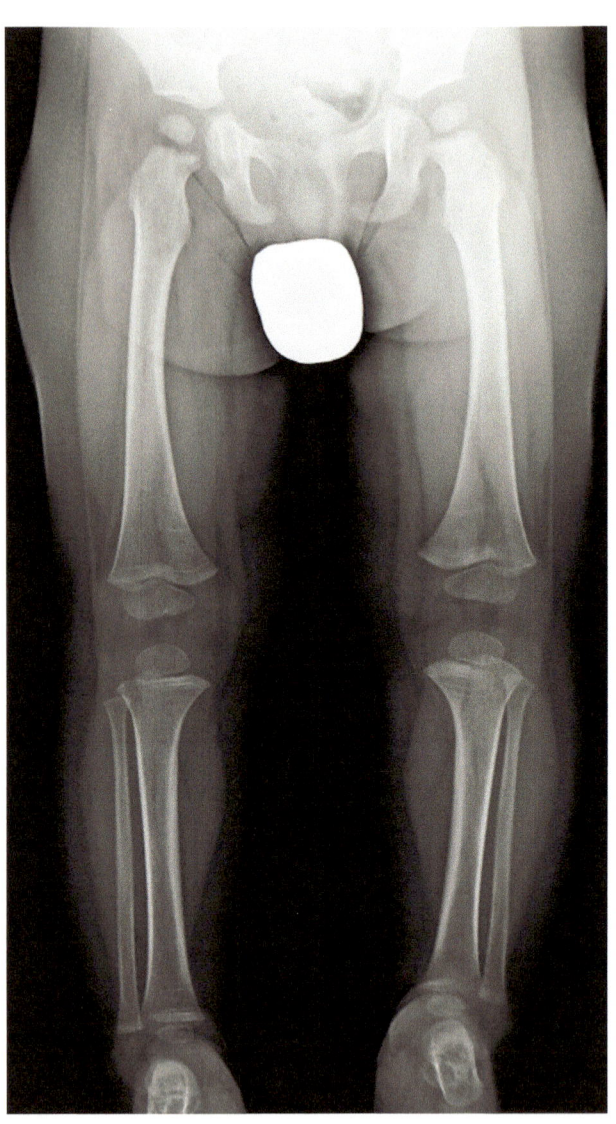

10

❓ Q2

Differential diagnosis includes:

(Multiple answers might be correct.)

1. Osteomyelitis
2. Acute arthritis
3. Eosinophilic granuloma
4. Blount disease (tibia vara)
5. Fibrous dysplasia

❓ Q3

Which of the following imaging techniques is the best to confirm the diagnosis?
(Only one option is correct.)

1. Bone scan
2. PET scan
3. CT with contrast media
4. MRI
5. CT without contrast media

❓ Q4
MRI was performed:

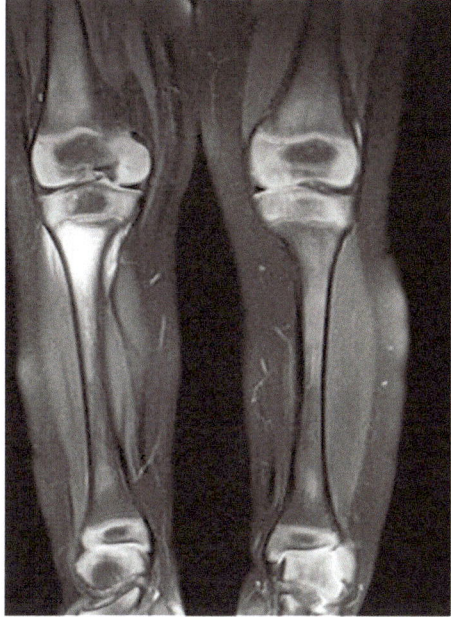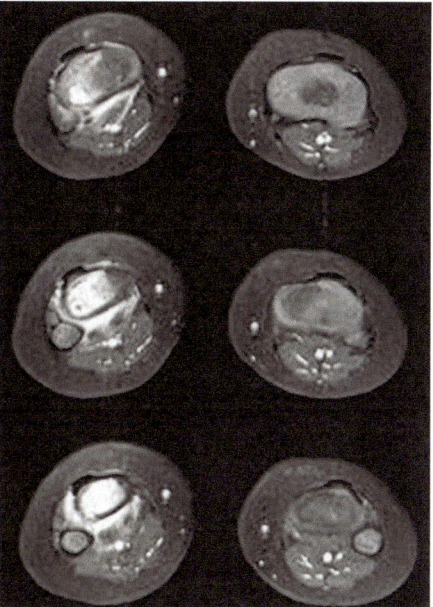

Give the most likely diagnosis.

_____

_____

_____

SC 2

A 3-year-old boy:
- Night headache for 3 weeks and acute vomiting last night at 3 AM
- Head CT was performed in emergency during night

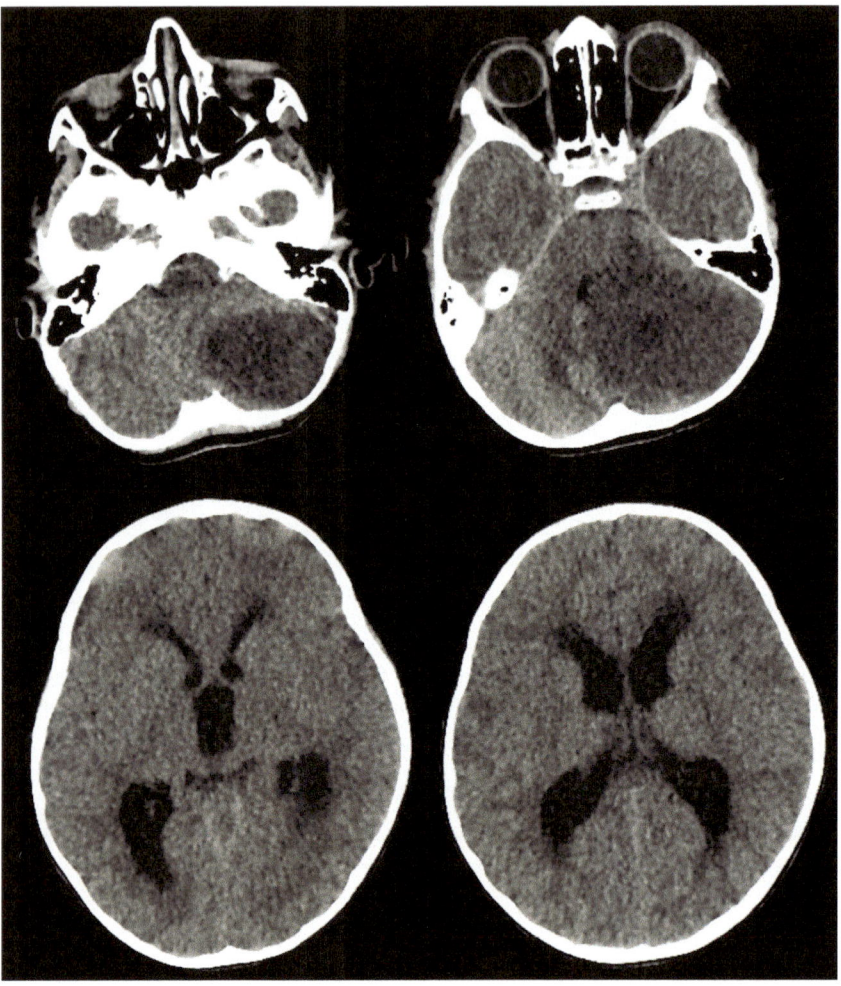

? **Q1**

Head CT was performed in emergency during night. Which of the following statements are correct?

(Multiple answers might be correct.)

1. Fourth ventricle is displaced by the mass
2. There is a mass within the left cerebellar hemisphere
3. Posterior CSF cisternae are occluded
4. Supratentorial ventricular system is dilated
5. The most likely diagnosis is a left cerebellar infarction

? Q2
What course of action would you take next?
(Multiple answers might be correct.)
1. Perform spinal MRI with contrast injection
2. Perform cerebral angiography
3. Perform head MRI with contrast injection
4. Perform head MRI without contrast injection
5. Perform lumbar CT

? Q3
MRI was performed after the CT:

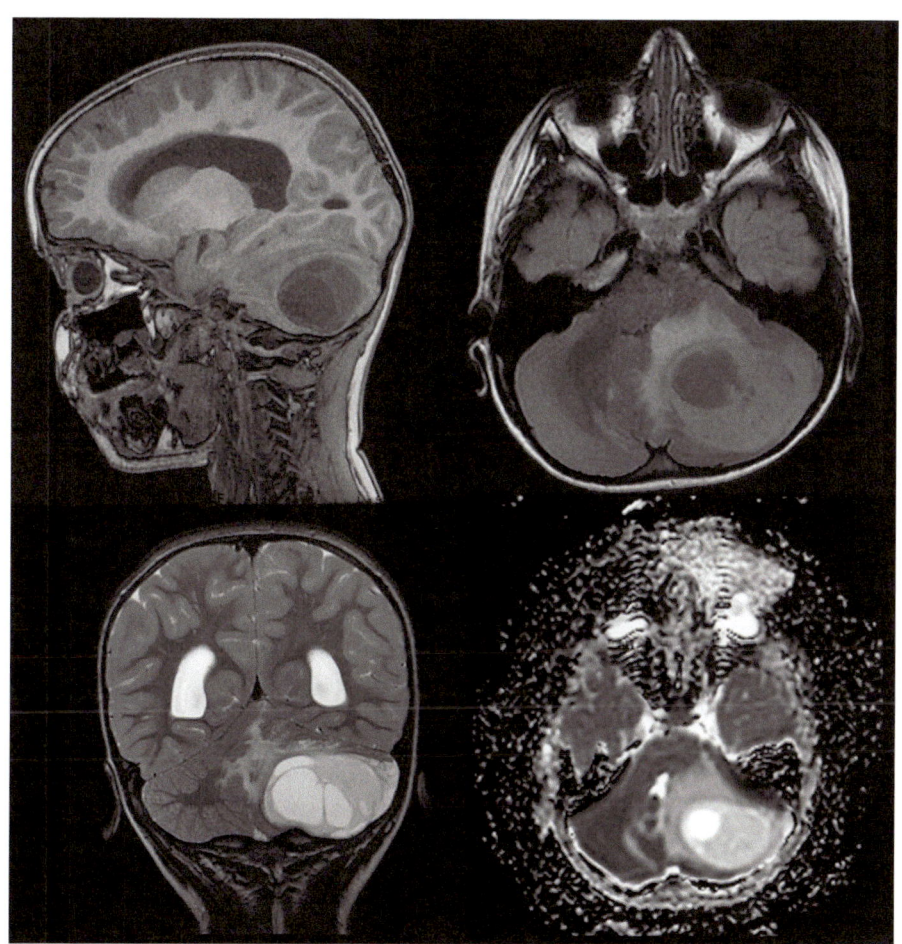

Which of the following statements are correct?
(Multiple answers might be correct.)

1. MRI demonstrates a cerebellar tumour
2. There is a water diffusion restriction within the solid part of the lesion
3. Head and spine MRI after contrast injection must be performed
4. Oedema is surrounding the lesion
5. The tumour exhibits a cystic component

? **Q4**

Head and spine MRI after contrast injection was also performed:

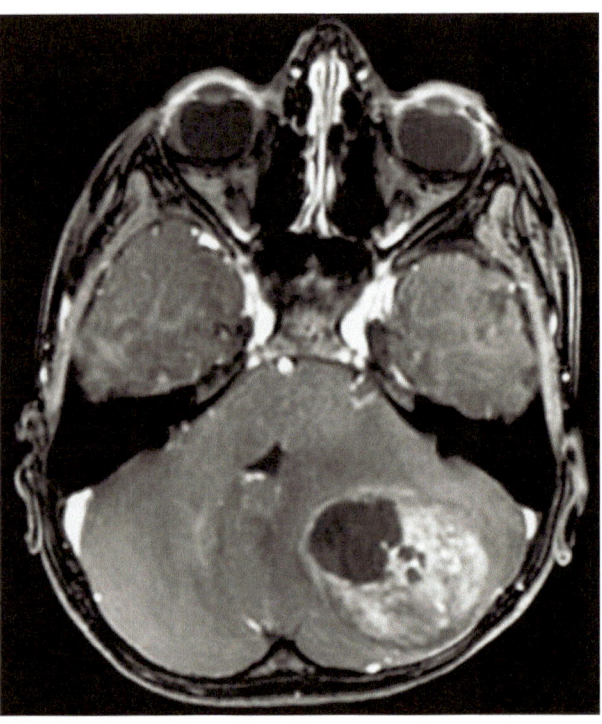

10

Differential diagnosis includes:
(Multiple answers might be correct.)

1. Medulloblastoma
2. Pilocytic astrocytoma
3. Neurofibroma
4. Ganglioglioma
5. Ependymoma

? Q5

Spine MRI was also performed:

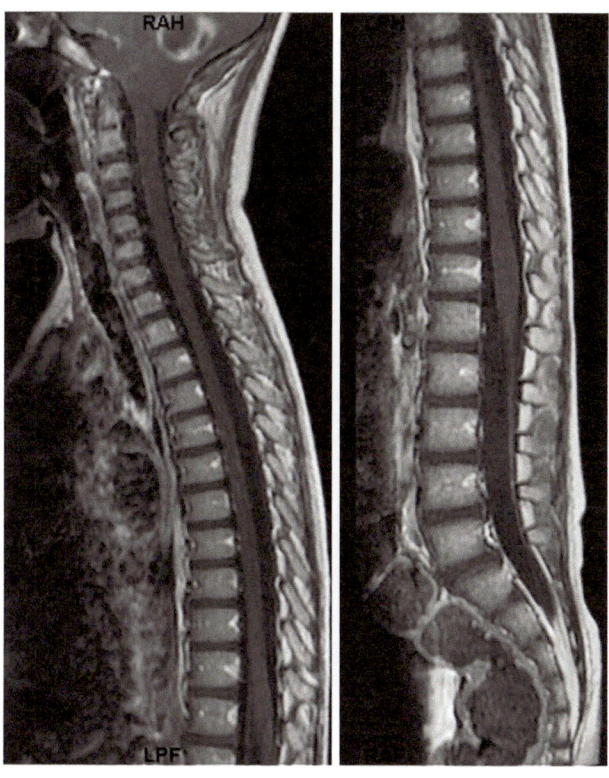

Give the most likely diagnosis.

_____

_____

_____

CORE

An 8-year-old girl:
— Presented with a painful left wrist after falling on an outstretched hand

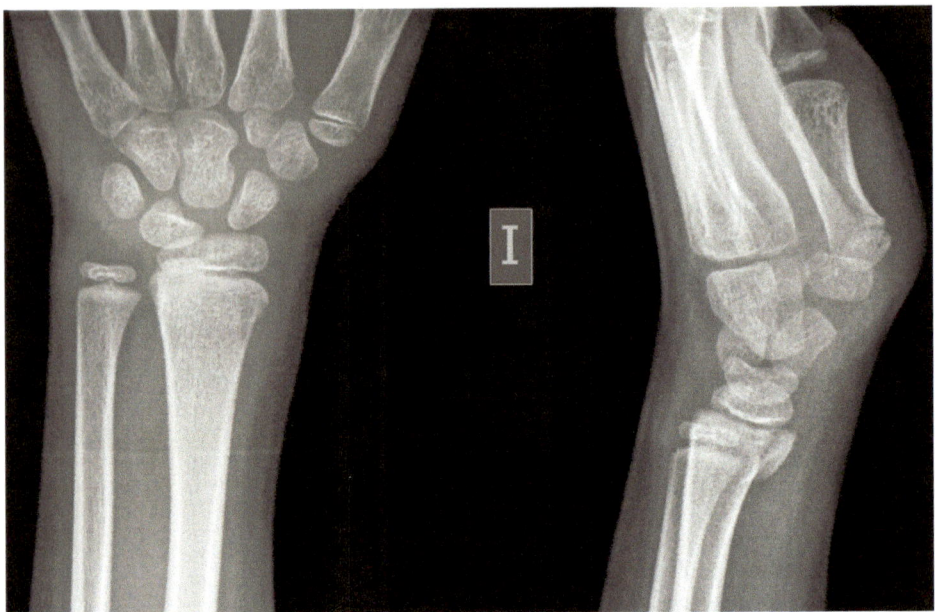

10

❓ Q1
Describe the relevant positive and negative findings.

_____

_____

_____

❓ Q2
Regarding this type of fracture in a child, indicate the correct answers.
(Multiple answers might be correct.)
1. Follow-up of at least 1 year is recommended
2. Premature physeal closure represents a possible complication
3. Partial involvement of the physis may lead to bone deformity
4. No follow-up is needed
5. Early follow-up within 5 days with X-ray is recommended

? Q3
List (at least) three potential sequelae and complications of these physeal injuries.

_____

_____

_____

Answers

Multiple Response Questions (MRQs)

✓ **MRQ 1**
1, 2, 4 and 5

✓ **MRQ 2**
1 and 4

✓ **MRQ 3**
1, 2 and 3

✓ **MRQ 4**
1, 2 and 5

✓ **MRQ 5**
1, 2, 4 and 5

Short Cases (SCs)

SC 1

✅ Q1

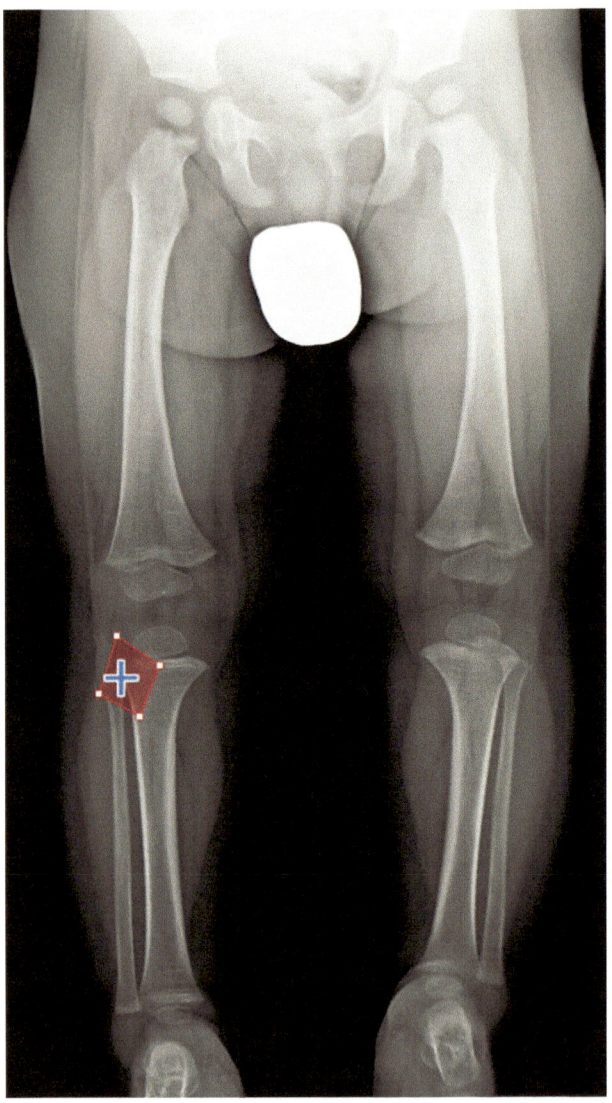

10

✅ Q2
1 and 3

✅ Q3
4

Q4

Subacute osteomyelitis (in relation with *Staphylococcus aureus*)

Explanation

Primary subacute epiphyseal and meta-epiphyseal osteomyelitis are frequent in toddlers. Radiological signs may not be present at the beginning of the infection. Lesion in most of the cases is close to the metaphyseal region. Swelling of the adjacent soft tissue can be observed.

SC 2

 Q1

1, 2, 3 and 4

✔ **Q2**

1 and 3

✔ **Q3**

1, 3, 4 and 5

✔ **Q4**

1 and 2

✔ **Q5**

Pilocytic astrocytoma

CORE

✔ **Q1**

Salter-Harris type II fracture of the distal radius (or an alternative detailed description: fracture line which involves the physis and metaphysis or fracture through the metaphysis of the distal radius which extends to the growth plate).

No significant/slight angulation or displacement is seen.

Explanation

It is important to identify the fracture, not to mistake normal growth plate for fracture, to appreciate normal alignment and provide information that would be relevant to the orthopaedic surgeon, like the involvement of the physis/growth plate in a child.

✔ **Q2**

1, 2, 3 and 5

Explanation

"During healing, growth arrest or growth acceleration may appear, secondary to physeal lesion. Partial Involvement of the physis or bone "bar" formation (between metaphysis and epiphysis) leads to bone end curvature. As a result, physeal bar resection may be required, or other surgical procedures may be necessary to prevent or correct deformity".

Q3

Residual angulation (alternatively state varus or valgus deformity), formation of bone bridges (also called bone bars), impaired growth (growth arrest), limb length discrepancies. Delayed complication: osteoarthritis.

As in any other fracture, problems with union (delayed union, non-union, pseudoarthrosis), osteomyelitis, arthritis.

Explanation

Physeal injuries are associated with disruption of the physis. Physeal discontinuity can focally disturb longitudinal growth. Bone bars (premature closure/ossification in some part of the physis) may result in angulations due to the remaining part of the bone which continues to grow. Intraarticular discontinuity in SH III and SH IV injuries may lead to early degenerative arthritis.

Literature

Adams A, Mankad K, Offiah C, Childs L. Branchial cleft anomalies: a pictorial review of embryological development and spectrum of imaging findings. Insights into Imaging. 2016;7(1):69–76.

Athanasakos A, Mazioti A, Economopoulos N, et al. Inflammatory bowel disease-the role of cross-sectional imaging techniques in the investigation of the small bowel. Insights into Imaging. 2015;6(1):73–83.

Charlotte de Lange. Radiology in paediatric non-traumatic thoracic emergencies. Insights into Imaging. 2011 October;2(5):585–98.

Cortazar AZ, Martín Martinez C, Duran Feliubadalo C, Bella Cueto MR, Serra L. Magnetic resonance imaging in the prenatal diagnosis of neural tube defects. Insights into Imaging. 2013;4(2):225–37.

Kakkar C, Kakkar S, Saggar K, Goraya JS, Ahluwalia A, Arora A. Paediatric brainstem: A comprehensive review of pathologies on MR imaging. Insights into Imaging. 2016;7(4):505–22.

Van Schuppen J, van Doorn Martine MAC, van Rijn Rick R. Childhood osteomyelitis: imaging characteristics. Insights into Imaging. 2012;3(5):519–33.

Young C, Xie C, Owens CM. Paediatric multi-detector row chest CT: what you really need to know. Insights into Imaging. 2012;3(3):229–46.

Additional EDiR Preparatory Materials

http://learn.myesr.org

EDiR Preparatory Sessions

http://learn.myesr.org
Congenital malformations of the brain.
Imaging of the pancreas.
Imaging of inflammatory bowel disease.

10

Safety in Radiology and Imaging Procedures

Multiple Response Questions (MRQs)

❓ MRQ 1
Because of the high risk of nephrogenic systemic fibrosis, which of the following gadolinium-based contrast agents is/are not recommended for use in a patient with end-stage renal failure?

(Multiple answers might be correct.)
1. Gadoteric acid (Dotarem)
2. Gadoteridol (ProHance)
3. Gadobutrol (Gadovist)
4. Gadodiamide (Omniscan)
5. Gadopentetic acid (Magnevist)

❓ MRQ 2
Regarding gadolinium as a contrast used in MRI, which of the following statements are correct?

(Multiple answers might be correct.)
1. Gadolinium-based contrast agents shorten the T1 relaxation times but not the T2
2. Unbound free gadolinium is extremely toxic and tends to be deposited in the liver, lymphatics and bones
3. The distribution of the gadolinium is limited to the intracellular space
4. Gadolinium is not visualised in CT
5. Gadolinium chelates are not metabolised in the body

❓ MRQ 3
Which of the following matchings between tracers/contrasts with their applications are correct?

(Multiple answers might be correct.)
1. Gadoteric acid (Dotarem) in biliary tree imaging
2. 18F-FDDNP in multiple sclerosis
3. Tc99m in Crohn's disease
4. 18F-FDG in lung cancer N staging
5. Gd-BOPTA in hepatocarcinoma (*MultiHance*)

❓ MRQ 4
Regarding safety considerations in the use of ionising radiation, which of the following sentences are correct?

(Multiple answers might be correct.)
1. Using grids with higher grid ratio decreases patient dose
2. It is safe for staff to stay near the patient provided the staff are not in the path of the primary beam
3. The DAP is a measure of the patient dose
4. In CT, the DLP decreases with scan length
5. Use of iterative reconstruction increases patient doses

? MRQ 5

Regarding safety considerations in ultrasound, which of the following sentences are correct?

(Multiple answers might be correct.)

1. Transient cavitation may lead to the formation of free radicals
2. Ultrasound-induced haemorrhage and lesions at lung surfaces are possible
3. Ultrasound under normal use is nonionising; therefore it is completely safe
4. Output power of the transducer is higher in Doppler than in B-mode imaging
5. The thermal index is an estimate of temperature rise at the transducer-skin interface

? MRQ 6

Regarding safety considerations in MRI, which of the following sentences are correct?

(Multiple answers might be correct.)

1. To avoid burns, one should instruct the patient not to touch the bore
2. Peripheral nerve stimulation in a motionless patient is produced by the static field
3. Cardiac pacemakers may be contraindicated depending on the type of device
4. The SAR is a measure of heat absorption in tissues
5. The main magnetic field is shut down after the last patient leaves, and it is therefore safe to bring ferromagnetic materials inside the MRI room

? MRQ 7

Regarding safety considerations in interventional procedures, which of the following sentences are correct?

(Multiple answers might be correct.)

1. Interventional procedures are relatively high radiation dose procedures
2. Eye lens injuries to staff are negligible
3. Staff work within the controlled area
4. Patient and radiologist doses are correlate
5. Image intensifier should be moved away from the patient for lower patient doses

Answers

Multiple Response Questions (MRQs)

MRQ 1

4 and 5

Explanation

Gadodiamide and gadopentetic acid. Linear GBCAs are considered the least stable and have been linked to most cases of the development of NSF. Estimated incidence for NSF in patients with severe renal failure is 3–18% after gadodiamide and 0.1–1% after gadopentetate dimeglumine.

The association between nephrogenic systemic fibrosis (NSF) and gadolinium-based contrast agents was recognised in 2006. Onset can be from the day of exposure for up to 2–3 months. Rarely, it can occur years after exposure. Early changes are pain, pruritus and swelling and erythema of the skin, which usually start in the legs. Later changes include fibrotic thickening of the skin, and subcutaneous tissues and limb contractures may occur. Fibrosis of internal organs, e.g. muscle, diaphragm, heart, liver and lungs, may also occur. There may be death if involvement of internal organs is severe.

The most important risk factor for development of NSF is the degree of renal dysfunction. The highest risk for development of NSF is seen in patients undergoing dialysis and those with severe (stage 4, glomerular filtration rate, 30–40 mL/min per 1.73 m2) or end-stage (stage 5, glomerular filtration rate < 30 mL/min per 1.73 m2) chronic kidney disease without dialysis or acute kidney injury.

The risk for NSF may be related to the type of GBCA chelate, cumulative dose and residual renal function of the patient. <u>Macrocyclic and ionic chelates tend to be more stable than other gadolinium compounds and, therefore, have a decreased risk for causing NSF.</u> **Linear GBCAs are considered the least stable and have been linked to most cases of the development of NSF. Estimated incidence for NSF in patients with severe renal failure is 3–18% after gadodiamide and 0.1–1% after gadopentetate dimeglumine.**

European Medicines Agency: Categorisation of GBCAs according to NSF risk, based on their thermodynamic and kinetic properties

I. **High risk (associated with greatest number of NSF cases)**
    A. Linear non-ionic chelates (gadoversetamide (OptiMARK™), gadodiamide (Omniscan®))
    B. Linear ionic chelates (gadopentetic acid (Magnevist®, Magnegita® and Gado-MRT-ratiopharm∗)
II. **Medium risk (associated with few, if any, unconfounded cases of NSF)**
    Linear ionic chelates
    Gadofosveset (Vasovist®), gadoxetic acid (Primovist®) and gadobenic acid (MultiHance®)
III. **Low risk (no renal function evaluation required before examination)**
    Macrocyclic chelates
    Gadoteric acid (Dotarem®), gadoteridol (ProHance®) and gadobutrol (Gadovist®)

✅ MRQ 2

2 and 5

Explanation

1. **Contrast agents containing Gd(III) shorten the observed longitudinal (T_1) and the transverse (T_2) relaxation time of water protons in their vicinity. In the body, water T2 is generally 5–20 times shorter than T1. As a result, the effect of a Gd(III) contrast agent will be much more pronounced on T1.** Because of this effect, Gd(III)-based agents are often referred to as T1-contrast agents because on a percentage basis they have a much larger effect on T1.

2. Gd3+ ions are of a similar size to calcium ions and competitively bind to numerous pharmacological targets, including voltage-gated calcium channels. Gadolinium ions are therefore complexed with chelating ligands to prevent toxicity when used in contrast media. Although the development of nephrogenic systemic fibrosis in patients with renal impairment is well documented, over recent years it has become apparent that exposure to GBCAs can potentially result in gadolinium deposition within human bone and brain tissue even in the presence of normal renal function.

3. These contrast agents are classified as extracellular fluid (ECF) contrast agents. They rapidly extravasate from the bloodstream into the tissue interstitial, extracellular spaces and are rapidly eliminated from the systemic circulation via filtration through the kidneys. Two of these agents (gadobenate disodium (Gd-BOPTA) and gadoxetate disodium (Gd-EOB-DTPA)) are partially excreted through the liver and into the bile and faeces.

4. Gadolinium, like iodine, is a heavy metal capable of attenuating X-rays. The atomic number of gadolinium ($Z = 64$) is higher than that of iodine ($Z = 53$). The k-edge of gadolinium is also more closely matched to the peak of the CT spectrum, meaning gadolinium absorbs a greater fraction of the X-ray beam than does iodine. However, the lower concentration and total number of gadolinium atoms administered in current formulations means that gadolinium contrast has a much lower visibility on CT than iodine contrast.

   (a) From the early 1990s to the mid-2000s, gadolinium contrast was occasionally used in CT and angiography in patients with severe allergies to iodinated contrast. With the recognition that high doses of gadolinium might precipitate nephrogenic systemic fibrosis, this technique was abandoned. Even today, a trace amount of contrast enhancement in the bladder or renal collecting systems may be noted in patients receiving a CT scan shortly after a gadolinium-enhanced MR study.

5. Gadolinium contrasts (GC) are not metabolised and are excreted by the kidneys. They distribute into the extracellular compartment. Because of its high intrinsic toxicity, gadolinium must be administered as a chelate. GC can be classified according to two key molecular features: (a) nature of the chelating moiety, either macrocyclic molecules in which gadolinium is caged in the pre-organised cavity of the ligand or linear, open-chain molecules, and (b) ionicity wherein Gd chelates can be ionic (meglumine or sodium salts) or non-ionic.

✅ MRQ 3

4 and 5

Explanation

1. The gadolinium chelates are mostly eliminated via the kidneys (including gadoteric acid), with some amount of liver excretion demonstrated for a few of the agents. Hepatobiliary-specific gadolinium agents include two of the high relaxivity agents: gadobenate disodium (Gd-BOPTA) and gadoxetate disodium (Gd-EOB-DTPA).

11

2. A brain MR imaging with gadolinium is recommended for the diagnosis of MS. A spinal cord MR imaging is recommended if the brain MR imaging is non-diagnostic or if the presenting symptoms are at the level of the spinal cord.

   (a) Positron emission tomography (PET) imaging with 2-(1-{6-[(2-[^{18}F]fluoro-ethyl)(methyl)amino]-2-naphthyl}ethylidene)malononitrile ([^{18}F]FDDNP) has been found useful to differentiate Alzheimer's disease (AD) from mild cognitive impairment (MCI) and normal ageing and to show prion protein amyloid accumulation in the brain of patients with Gerstmann–Sträussler–Scheinker (GSS) disease. [^{18}F]FDDNP is currently the only PET molecular imaging probe known to label both amyloid and tangles in the living brain.

3. Statement 1.8. ECCO-ESGAR Diagnostics GL (2018) patients with clinical suspicion of CD and with normal endoscopy should be considered for small bowel capsule endoscopy (SBCE) evaluation or cross-sectional imaging. If stenotic disease is suspected, risk of retention should be assessed.

4. ^{18}F-fluorodeoxyglucose positron emission tomography (FDG-PET) is critical for staging non-small-cell lung cancer (NSCLC). ^{18}F-2-deoxy-D-glucose (FDG) positron emission tomography (PET scan) has become a standard tool for determining the operative candidacy of individuals with lung cancer by evaluating for the presence of regional or systemic metastases. FDG is a fluorescent glucose analogue that accumulates at sites with elevated glucose metabolism, including many tumours. It has been well established that the degree of FDG uptake by NSCLC tumours (i.e. the intensity) predicts survival, even among early-stage surgical candidates.

5. The diagnosis of HCC is primarily based on noninvasive standard imaging methods, such as ultrasound (US), dynamic multiphasic multidetector-row CT (MDCT) and magnetic resonance imaging (MRI). Some experts advocate gadolinium diethylenetriamine pentaacetic acid (Gd-EOB-DTPA) MRI and contrast-enhanced US as the promising imaging modalities of choice.

   (a) The gadolinium chelates are mostly eliminated via the kidneys, with some amount of liver excretion demonstrated for a few of the agents. Hepatobiliary-specific gadolinium agents include two of the high relaxivity agents: gadobenate disodium (Gd-BOPTA) and gadoxetate disodium (Gd-EOB-DTPA).

✓ **MRQ 4**

3

Explanation

1. Higher grid ratios increase the clean-up of scattered photons, but they also stop some primary image-forming photons from reaching the detector. Therefore, for there to be sufficient photons to form the image, the mAs is increased leading to a higher patient dose.

2. The member of staff will receive a dose from the photons scattered off the patient and falling on him/her.

3. In projection radiography, DAP stands for dose area product. It is derived from the intensity of the X-ray beam and the area of the patient irradiated and is a measure of the total amount of energy falling on the patient and therefore patient dose.

4. The DLP is proportional to the length of patient scanned.
5. Wise use of iterative reconstruction can reduce patient dose without reducing the image quality.

MRQ 5
1, 2 and 4
Explanation
1. Transient cavitation leads to small points of very high temperature leading to breaking of chemical bonds and therefore free radicals.
2. This is because of the stress that focused ultrasound imposes on the lung's air–blood barrier.
3. There are mechanical and thermal bio-effects of ultrasound. Since their effects are not totally known or understood, it is important to use ultrasound prudently by avoiding unnecessary scanning.
4. Since we require echoes from blood components (red blood cells) and such echoes are small, we need to transmit at higher powers for an adequate signal.
5. It is an estimate of temperature rise inside the body.

MRQ 6
1, 3 and 4
Explanation
1. This avoids sparks between the patient and bore surface.
2. This is produced by the rapidly changing gradient fields not the static field.
3. The strong magnetic field or gradients would impact the functioning of the device. Having said this all pacemaker vendors now offer MRI-compatible pacemakers.
4. SAR stands for specific absorption rate, which is a measure of the radiation energy changed to heat in the patient. This would lead to temperature rise within the patient.
5. The static field is never off!

MRQ 7
1, 3 and 4
Explanation
1. Interventional procedures are often long and complex and done under image guidance hence leading to high patient stochastic and skin doses.
2. Although the interventionist should never be in the primary beam, scatter from the patient reaches his/her eyes. It is important to wear eye protective goggles.
3. The X-ray room where the patient is imaged is a controlled area (high dose area). The interventionist and other healthcare professionals work within this area and not behind a protective cubicle. Protective apparel such as lead gowns are therefore mandatory.
4. The higher the amount of radiation falling on the patient, the higher the amount of scatter from the patient falling on the interventionist.
5. When the image intensifier is moved away from the patient, the inverse square law dictates that the intensity of radiation falling on it decreases. To maintain the image quality constant, the intensity of the primary beam has to be increased by increasing the mA, hence leading to higher patient dose.

Literature

European Society of Radiology. White paper on radiation protection by the European Society of Radiology. Insights Imaging. 2011;2:357–62.

Häusler U, Czarwinski R, Brix G. Radiation exposure of medical staff from interventional x-ray procedures: a multicentre study. European Radiology. 2009;19(8):2000–8.

Jakobsen JÅ, Oyen R, Thomsen HS, Morcos SK. Safety of ultrasound contrast agents. European Radiology. 2005;15(5):941–5.

Khawaja AZ, Cassidy DB, Al Shakarchi J, McGrogan DG, Inston NG, Jones RG. Revisiting the risks of MRI with Gadolinium based contrast agents—review of literature and guidelines. Insights Imaging. 2015;6:553–8.

Shulman RM, Hunt B. Cardiac implanted electronic devices and MRI safety in 2018—the state of play. Eur Radiol. 2018;28(10):4062–5.

Additional EDiR Preparatory Materials

http://learn.myesr.org

11

Principles of Imaging Techniques and Processing

© European Board of Radiology (EBR) 2019
J. Babar et al., *EDiR - The Essential Guide*, https://doi.org/10.1007/978-3-030-20066-4_12

Multiple Response Questions (MRQs)

? MRQ 1
Regarding general digital radiography, which of the following sentences are correct?
(Multiple answers might be correct.)
1. A more penetrating X-ray beam has a lower percentage of high-energy photons
2. Differential linear attenuation coefficient of tissues makes X-ray imaging possible
3. Scatter increases dose to non-imaged organs
4. Limiting spatial resolution is a function of both focal spot size and detector pixel size
5. Increasing the kV decreases the image contrast between tissues

? MRQ 2
Regarding ultrasound imaging, which of the following sentences are correct?
(Multiple answers might be correct.)
1. Reflection is high at the interface between tissues of similar acoustic impedance
2. dB is the unit of acoustic impedance
3. Acoustic impedance is the product of density and frequency
4. The wavelength of the ultrasound beam is equal to the thickness of the piezo-electric crystal
5. Absorption of ultrasound in tissues results in heat production

? MRQ 3
Regarding CT, which of the following sentences are correct?
(Multiple answers might be correct.)
1. mA modulation leads to more uniform image quality
2. There is a linear relationship between CT number and attenuation coefficient of tissues
3. CT produces high-contrast images because it reduces production of scatter in the patient
4. Higher pitch leads to higher patient doses
5. The value of the CT number (in Hounsfield units) for water is 0

? MRQ 4
Regarding MRI, which of the following sentences are correct?
(Multiple answers might be correct.)
1. The patient is placed in the main field, and a fraction of the protons align with the main magnetic field to form a net tissue magnetisation vector (M)
2. The Larmor frequency is independent of the strength of the main field
3. In T1-weighted images, the higher the water content, the brighter is the tissue
4. The T1 of water is around 500 ms
5. Cortical bone exhibits a very low signal intensity in conventional MR images because of its very short T2

12

❓ MRQ 5

Regarding PET, which of the following sentences are correct?
(Multiple answers might be correct.)
1. It has a lower detection sensitivity than gamma camera imaging
2. Radionuclides chosen should have positrons emitted with low ranges in tissues
3. Lower-quality CT images are often acceptable
4. F-18 decays to O-18 and positron with a half-life of 109.6 mins
5. Radiation protection of staff is less difficult than gamma camera imaging

Answers

Multiple Response Questions (MRQs)

✅ MRQ 1

2, 3, 4 and 5
Explanation
1. High-energy photons are more penetrating unlike low-energy photons which are easily attenuated.
2. Digital radiography (and CT) measure linear attenuation coefficient of tissues and then attach a corresponding greyscale level to the corresponding pixel. Hence if all tissues had the same linear attenuation coefficient, the image would be a single greyscale level throughout!
3. Photons are scattered by tissues (mostly by Compton interaction) in all directions within the patient including out of the direction of the incident beam. They may fall and be absorbed anywhere including within radiosensitive tissues which are not in the volume irradiated by the incident beam. Hence the increased dose.
4. Limiting spatial resolution (also known as line-pair resolution) is the maximum line-pair frequency (in line-pairs per mm) that can be visualised clearly. A large focal spot produces blurring, and hence line-pairs will be blurred and close ones not seen. Similarly, if the size of a detector pixel is large, for example, higher than the width of a line-pair, the latter will not be seen.
5. As one moves towards higher kVs, the difference in linear attenuation coefficient between tissues decreases, and hence the image contrast also decreases.

✅ MRQ 2

1
Explanation
1. The higher the difference in acoustic impedance between two tissues (e.g. bone/soft tissue, soft tissue/air), the higher the reflection.
2. dB is always related to a RATIO of two values of the same variable (intensities, powers, etc). Acoustic impedance is the product (not ratio) of tissue density and ultrasound velocity (two different variables).
3. Acoustic impedance is defined as the product of tissue density and ultrasound velocity in the tissue.

4. The thickness of the crystal is equal to HALF of the wavelength of the ultrasound wave.
5. As the tissues vibrate under the action of the ultrasound beam, one can consider that viscosity/frictional force effects within/between sections of the tissue convert the ultrasound energy into heat.

✅ MRQ 3
1, 2 and 5
Explanation
1. If one were to maintain a constant mA all along the patient's body, thick body sections would lead to low penetration, and therefore a high level of noise in the image as the number of photons reaching the detectors is low (conversely with thin body parts). Modulation increases the mA in thick areas of the patient automatically in an attempt to maintain noise levels constant throughout the scan.
2. The equation relating CT number and attenuation coefficient of tissues is a linear equation. A graph of CT number of tissue on the y-axis and attenuation coefficient of tissues on the x-axis is linear.
3. CT does not reduce the amount of scatter produced in the patient, but it does reduce the amount of scatter reaching the detector.
4. Patient-dose increases as pitch decreases as there is more overlap of slices.
5. This follows directly from the equation defining the CT number.

✅ MRQ 4
1 and 5
Explanation
1. True the patient protons need to be aligned with the main magnetic field and form a net tissue magnetisation (M) vector, so that they can be induced to emit signals by the measuring (excitation) pulse.
2. The Larmor frequency is proportional to the strength of the main static field.
3. Water has very long T1 relaxation time; it has the lowest signal amplitude on T1-weighted images because there is a low recovery of the M vector over the TR period.
4. T1 of water is around 3000ms.
5. Cortical bone has low T2 arising from the fact that it is low in water content, and calcium does not produce an MRI signal because its spin quantum number is zero.

✅ MRQ 5
2, 3 and 4
Explanation
1. The absence of large collimators in PET increases the number of photons reaching the detectors; fewer image-forming photons are lost leading to higher sensitivity.
2. This is important to ensure that the point where the positron is annihilated and from where the back-to-back photons are emitted is close to the actual location of the FDG. If the range is long, then the spatial information would be incorrect.

3. CT images for PET often play a secondary function, which is to be able to better identify the location within the tissues where the FDG has been deposited. In such cases, the images do not always need to be full diagnostic quality CT images.
4. This is the half-life of F-18.
5. Radiation protection of staff is more difficult as the photon energies in PET are much higher and therefore more penetrating than those in gamma imaging.

Literature

Beyer T, Townsend DW, Czernin J, Freudenberg LS. The future of hybrid imaging - part 2: PET/CT. Insights into Imaging. 2011;2(3):225–34.

Eshed I, Krabbe S, Østergaard M, et al. Influence of field strength, coil type and image resolution on assessment of synovitis by unenhanced MRI – a comparison with contrast-enhanced MRI. European Radiology. 2015;25(4):1059–67.

Evans A, Trimboli RM, Athanasiou A, Balleyguier C, et al. Breast ultrasound: recommendations for information to women and referring physicians by the European Society of Breast Imaging. Insights into Imaging. 2018;9(4):449–61.

Kotter E, Langer M. Digital radiography with large-area flat-panel detectors. Eur Radiol. 2002;12: 2562–70.

Lechel U, Becker C, Langenfeld-Jäger G, Brix G. Dose reduction by automatic exposure control in multidetector computed tomography: comparison between measurement and calculation. European Radiology. 2009;19(4):1027–34.

Additional EDiR Preparatory Materials

http://learn.myesr.org

Management

© European Board of Radiology (EBR) 2019
J. Babar et al., *EDiR - The Essential Guide*, https://doi.org/10.1007/978-3-030-20066-4_13

Multiple Response Questions (MRQs)

 MRQ 1

In relation to the errors/discrepancies in radiology, which of the following statements are correct?
(Multiple answers might be correct.)
1. The errors/discrepancies in radiology are both inevitable and avoidable
2. The errors of radiologists occur only derived of the human factor
3. Strategies exist to minimise error causes and to learn from errors made
4. The use of structured reporting has been advocated as an error reduction strategy
5. The use of CAD has a role in minimising the likelihood of missing some radiologic abnormalities

Answers

Multiple Response Questions (MRQs)

 MRQ 1
1, 3, 4 and 5

Literature

Brady AP. Error and discrepancy in radiology: inevitable or avoidable? Insights into Imaging. 2017;8(1):171–82.
European Society of Radiology (ESR). ESR guidelines for the communication of urgent and unexpected findings. Insights into Imaging. 2012;3(1):1–3.
European Society of Radiology (ESR). The ESR Audit Tool (Esperanto): genesis, contents and pilot. Insights into Imaging. 2018;9(6):899–903.

13

Additional EDiR Preparatory Materials

http://learn.myesr.org